The Wellness Seed

An inspirational wellness story bringing emotional and practical support on the cancer journey.

Hillary Polednik

COPYRIGHT

Disclaimer

The information provided in this book is not a substitute for medical treatment or professional advice. The author makes no legal claims, and the material is not intended to replace the services of a certified healthcare practitioner.

The information provided reflects a good faith effort to be accurate but cannot be guaranteed as to accuracy. Regarding information that expresses an opinion (e.g. ranking or a recommended course of action), such information expresses only an opinion based on the practical experience of persons who do not hold themselves as experts on the matters covered.

This book is dedicated to

Rudolf John Polednik and Rudolf Milan Polednik

CONTENTS

INTRODUCTION

We carry inside us
the wonders
we seek outside us.

- Rumi

INTRODUCTION

Embrace who you are, where you came from, what you are here
to do and how to take advantage of every opportunity along the
way. Manage grief, tune into your own healing, find forgiveness,
enhance your intuition, hear your own guidance from the spirit
world, establish powerful relationships.

- James Van Praagh, *Talking to Heaven*

I was diagnosed with Stage 2 estrogen-positive breast cancer in June
2011 just before my 45th birthday. I found the small lump in the
shower one morning. I had been in for a routine mammogram but
I did not catch the tumor due to the high position and location. I had
two lumpectomy surgeries in late June and during the same time,
an infected tooth from a root canal pulled in July. In August, I began
chemotherapy and then radiation in January.

You hear many stories about how cancer impacts people's lives, but
before I was diagnosed, I never understood it. I was curious and
used to wonder what it was like for someone going through cancer.
My experience has been profound on so many levels that I have been
compelled to write about it, first because of the Wellness Project
that came out of it, and second, to share my personal perspective
which I hope will be valuable for you on your journey.

The seed of the Wellness Project originated in the infusion room
at the local hospital where I was undergoing treatment. One day,
about two months into chemotherapy, a group of women and I were
sitting together talking. "Why did we get cancer?" someone asked.
"What are the root causes? And what are we specifically doing to get
well besides chemotherapy?" From there, we started sharing

"alternative" resource ideas for cancer treatment, including acupuncture, massage, nutrition, supplements, energy healing, meditation, and visualization practices.

These approaches didn't replace conventional treatments like surgery, chemotherapy and radiation, but we discovered they were essential complements. One woman who was sitting across from me announced, "I'm not in a position to write these alternative health tips down but someone needs to put all this knowledge together."

Here we were, four women sitting in the infusion room together on brown leather recliner chairs attached to chemotherapy drips. Each one of us had received a collection of lengthy health books and cookbooks from friends and family with good intentions to read but we just couldn't manage to get through all the books with everything else on our immediate plates.

I knew at that exact moment that I was the person who could streamline all the health information to create the Wellness Project. This information would not just be a memoir but would include a collection of wellness tips, mindset tips, websites, books, and various wellness resources as well as real-life stories and experiences with cancer. I would include my alternative practitioners whose treatments alleviated my symptoms, stories about friends as well as writing and reflections about cancer from the heart.

After finishing seven months of treatment, I met with two friends, Betsy and Jennifer, at Betsy's home to discuss our health and wellness ideas for a website. Betsy was a registered nurse and Jennifer was a designer and worked in the field of integrative and functional nutrition. We had a common purpose, as we had each experienced family health challenges which we wanted to share with each other.

Betsy had a daughter who was born with a rare cancer and Jennifer had celiac, an autoimmune condition and a young son on the autism spectrum. We envisioned putting together a health and wellness directory and website of information to inspire people to get well again and reach a path of health restoration. This was not just going to be a dry list. The goal was to make the resources as useful as possible. We listed everything in the scope of our Wellness Project from early symptoms data information to an on-line wellness board to numerous wellness resources based in San Francisco. This was the first step of what would become The Wellness Seed.

I wrote this book to share my experiences and reflections that grew out of my healing process from cancer. I also wanted to simplify all the wellness information out there in the world and provide ideas and resources from my own journal and healing process to help others with their recovery. As I was seeking meaningful significance and purpose in my own life, I wanted to make a difference in the world and reassure others. I also believe the people and stories I encountered will provide insights for the caregiver who walks the healing path with his or her loved one.

PART I

DIAGNOSIS & TREATMENT

When the crucial beliefs that have created the blockage
in a healthy, forward flow to life are discovered and dislodged,
the full energy of life can flow smoothly once again.
And with that flow can come the vital force that will restore
the body's natural defenses to normal potency.

- O. Carl Simonton, MD, Getting Well Again

Chapter 1

WHAT HAPPENS WHEN YOU GET A CANCER DIAGNOSIS

I found the lump in the shower one morning in the middle of May 2011. This lump was located very high up in my left breast cavity at about 12 o'clock. It was the size of a small pebble and you could visibly see it protruding from under my skin when I put my arm behind my back. I showed my husband in the kitchen after getting out of the shower one morning and he said, "Go get that checked out."

So, I made an appointment to see my OBGYN doctor in late May. This appointment went smoothly. My OBGYN did not initially believe this little hard lump was anything to be alarmed about but he recommended a biopsy. The biopsy appointment did not happen straight away, as I was shortly flying to Florida to see my mother for a week with my two young children, Anna (age 7) and Tomas (age 5). I remember during this trip intuitively knowing something was just not right. You have to listen to your body and to your intuition. Not only was I more tired than usual, but I had also dropped significant weight for no apparent reason and I had a distracting ache in my back behind my back left collar bone. Additionally, my gum on the upper left side inside of my mouth just above the tooth where I had an old root canal was now pink and inflamed.

When I returned to San Francisco from my Florida trip in the middle of June, I had a biopsy and breast ultrasound. This procedure took some time with nurses coming in and out of the room. The process was hush-hush, and not much was communicated. The two nurses acted very professionally, were busy taking snapshots and looking at the monitor. I left not knowing anything except that there was "this lump."

I was at the local playground with my son Tomas when I received the call from Dr. Filler, my long-time OBGYN. Dr. Filler is a witty and heartfelt man. He delivered both my children by c-section at our local San Francisco hospital and he felt like family. Every year I sent him a holiday card and a newsy note. "We need to talk," he said. "The biopsy result came back as cancer."

I immediately started to cry and I kept crying for a few minutes as I sat in the park that day with my son. News that you have cancer is quite shocking. In the past, I used to think cancer happened to other people and I never imagined it would or could ever happen to me. As I was pretty shaken, the nurse on the phone asked me if I had support at home and I assured her I did as my husband, children, family and friends would be there for me.

What was a surprise that I did not anticipate was the high anxiety, panic and fear that kicked in straight after I received the diagnosis. Just two days later, I was aware of a constant clicking, a popping noise in my right ear and I convinced myself that not only did I have breast cancer but I might also have a brain tumor. I told my husband I was going to the local grocery store to pick up a couple of items as I did not want to alarm him--but instead, I walked up the hill from my apartment in San Francisco to the nearby Emergency room and checked myself in.

The doctor on duty that day must have known I was suffering from high anxiety when I told him I had just received a breast cancer diagnosis a few days beforehand. After taking my blood pressure and temperature and asking me a couple of clarifying questions that ruled out brain cancer, he prescribed an anti-anxiety medication. I had never taken anti-anxiety medication before so the feeling was one I will never forget. You could have told me a meteor was headed towards earth, directly towards San Francisco, and I would have taken it all in stride.

However, one of the side effects was fatigue. I was so exhausted by the afternoon I could not keep my eyes open and had to take a nap. I remember visiting my friend Daphne with my family at her house for dinner in Marin and I asked her if I could lay down in her bedroom before dinner as I was so tired. After a few days, I didn't like the fatigue side effect so I stopped taking the medication. The one thing I found that did help with my anxiety during this time was walking and I did a lot of walking up and down the hills in San Francisco to calm down and clear my mind.

The next few weeks were a whirlwind blur. My lumpectomy surgery was scheduled for June 22, 2011. This went smoothly. After the surgery, I recovered up in Calistoga at Indian Springs resort where I relaxed in the natural thermal mineral pool and celebrated my 45th birthday with my husband and children. On June 28 I had a second operation to clear the margins. Gratefully, I only had one lymph node removed. Because one lymph node was involved the cancer cells could travel to other areas of my body. My oncologist let me know this meant three months of chemotherapy and two months of radiation treatment to kill off any fast-growing cancer cells that may have spread to other locations of my body amongst the regular, normal cells.

On July 3, 2011, my whole extended family flew to Honolulu for the week to celebrate my mother-in-law's 70th birthday which was a nice family gathering despite the situation I was preparing to face mentally and physically with chemotherapy looming on my arrival back home. On July 29 I had my tooth from an old root canal pulled which now had an infected gum. This extraction had to happen before chemotherapy started as my immune system could not be compromised during the healing process.

I was about to start chemotherapy and felt very emotional. I shed a lot of tears as I confronted and began to release the stuffed emotions and past chapters in my life. I was finally addressing and processing the grief of my father's passing. I was also grieving the sadness of not being able to attend my niece's wedding on August 27, in Hanover, New Hampshire where my daughter was to be her flower girl.

Chapter 2

UPS AND DOWNS

The wound is the place where the Light enters you.

- Rumi

I really did not know what to expect from my first chemo treatment. I had been in the hospital previously and sat in a small room with a nurse practitioner for a tutorial session called, "chemo teach," where you learn about what to expect, including the typical side effects. You never quite know how the chemotherapy is going to react in your own individual system as everyone responds differently and nothing quite prepares you for the treatment phase. I listened to the instruction, asked a few questions and took notes.

My husband, Rudi joined me on the fifth floor of the local San Francisco hospital for my first chemo as moral support and to hold my hand. I had a water bottle and some magazines with me in a bag as I was told it was a three-hour session to receive the infusion. I remember I was calm but a bit nervous as I walked into the unknown. The whole experience felt bizarre.

First I got weighed in and my blood pressure taken by one of the nurses. I was led into one of the small infusion rooms to a comfortable leather recliner and given anti-nausea medication to swallow. The nurse put an IV into a vein in my left forearm and went to get my chemotherapy bags and then shortly returned. The first chemo bag was hung on a hook above my chair and dripped down into my IV.

The nurses were very caring, thoughtful and explained everything as they went along. They spoke gently to me which put me at ease with all the uncertainty. I worked at relaxing, breathing, and using the visualization technique my practitioner, Jumbe, had taught me in Acupuncture. I looked at Rudi's gentle face and held his hand. The other women around me receiving chemotherapy were either resting or asleep in their recliners, reading or talking quietly to their loved ones. A nurse assigned to me checked in to see how I was doing. After a while, I felt drowsy and fell asleep. I got up to use the restroom twice because my bladder was so full of fluid from the infusion and the water I was continuously drinking. I had to walk carefully to the restroom with the chemotherapy station attached on rollers and connected to the IV in my arm and then carefully maneuver and roll the station back to the side of my leather recliner.

After treatment, I walked across the street with Rudi to the parking garage. I was mentally groggy and had to use the restroom urgently again but there wasn't one close by. I looked around and considered my options. As embarrassing as it was at the time, I rushed behind a parked car and let it all flow out. Gratefully, besides my husband, nobody saw this faux pas.

Eight days after I started chemo I shaved my hair off at a local hair salon with Rudi and a few friends surrounding me for emotional support. This was a practical choice to bring control to a delicate time as I did not want to see all my hair fall out on my pillow.

Unexpected Intimacy

Over several chemo sessions, I became used to the infusion process and seeing all the familiar faces. It was an intimate time sitting alongside all these new friends and I felt happy. You could feel the oneness. I would describe this oneness as a state of being completely united with someone or something, an awareness you feel in your heart. These women around me were going through a similar experience, sharing similar feelings. We would commiserate about similar symptoms or circumstances we were facing and share tips and suggestions on what was working for us to combat the symptoms. As a community, we felt grounded. We were an extension of one another with the commonalities of our shared experience. I enjoyed the feeling of bonding and the friendships that were created.

During this time I also became close with two of my infusion nurses, Jeannie and Elona. They both looked after me during my sessions with ongoing care and kindness and provided emotional support and friendship.

Shift in Consciousness
How can I describe this shift in consciousness from before I received the cancer diagnosis to after I received the cancer diagnosis?

Five years before cancer I was living with a different state of mind. I was doing the best I could day-to-day caring for a baby and a toddler who were 23 months apart while my husband was often traveling for business. I was also preoccupied with my parents' lives as my father was very sick living with a neurological disease in a nursing home in Florida. My father's disease was complicated and was never officially diagnosed even by the top doctors at Mayo Clinic.

My father had moved from our family home in Florida into a nursing facility for round the clock care as he was deteriorating physically and mentally from a neurological disease. He could not walk with his walker any longer and he was in a wheelchair or in bed throughout the day watching DVDs. He had a catheter full time and was suffering from urinary tract infections from the catheter and abscesses from lying in the same position in bed.

I was my mother and father's daily sounding board on the phone. Every day I called and heard all about their day. There were small joyful moments such as my father receiving a letter or package but there were also, of course, the trials and tribulations. As a cancer sign and empath, I was absorbing their emotional upset like a sponge. I felt helpless and stressed out. I was living across the country caring for my children and I felt bad that I was not able to be in Florida to help them. With his continued physical challenges and neurological decline, my father decided to stop eating and with this decision soon after passed away March 23, 2006, at the age of 79 just five years before my cancer diagnosis.

After my father's death, I forged on with my day-to-day not properly grieving his passing. Then suddenly in what felt like a blink of an eye I'm the one diagnosed with cancer. This is when my shift in consciousness began. The first thing I consciously decided to do with encouragement from my friend Amy was to slow down. I would describe the feeling as a letting go process. I chose to come off autopilot from my familiar day-to-day rushing around. I started to truly appreciate and pay close attention to all the small joyful moments in each day such as holding my children's hands walking to school, reading in my son's kindergarten classroom, sitting in our dining room observing the hummingbirds fly between red flowers in the trees across the street or watching and listening to the wild San Francisco parrots fly overhead.

I was more aware of being in the moment and felt more happiness as I was having deep and meaningful conversations with friends and family. Despite what was going on externally, I felt more centered internally. Consciously working on changing old habits and beliefs, I decided to dig deep within myself, stay grounded and steer a steady course. I was going through a process of giving up control, surrendering and trusting that everything would turn out okay. I discovered you have to be okay with your new normal not knowing what is going to happen next but have faith that whatever that next is, it will turn out for the best and everything will be alright.

I was really blown open through cancer to see all the beauty around me because I was brought down physically to the depths of the pond and I felt all this light above me. I was in a pure conscious state and became acutely aware of everything that was happening within me and around me. There were emotional ups and downs and times when I would feel sorry for myself and got down in the dumps about how I felt and looked but my overall feeling was contentment. Cancer is a stepping stone process. It's about taking one day at a time and one step in front of the other. The truth is that being diagnosed with cancer is not something you wish for yourself or for others but perhaps it teaches important lessons, heartfelt understanding of the realistic hardships that unfold in life, and the ability to deepen into your true nature.

Chapter 3

MY TREATMENT SCHEDULE

Let Difficulty transform you. And it will.
In my experience, we just need help in learning
how not to run away.

- Pema Chodron

I started chemotherapy on August 18, 2011. Just three days
previously, my daughter had started second grade and my son had
started Kindergarten—so the daily task of getting organized took
on new meaning with my cancer treatment schedule. I created an
email group of friends and family to help manage the logistics and
keep everyone updated on my progress. I also kept a journal to
capture the experience. Throughout the chaos, Rudi and my close
friends, Laura and Jennifer made me smile and laugh, all the while
lifting my spirits with their kindness and support.

UPDATE EMAILS

August 13, 2011

I am feeling positive and trying to take this one day at a time. I
honestly feel a lot better since the operations and seeing my
nutritionist. Many have asked about the results from my Oncotype.
The Oncotype examines a patient's breast cancer tumor tissue at
a molecular level, determining how 21 specific genes, 16 genes
linked to breast cancer and 5 control genes, are expressed. The
measurement of these genes is calculated to give an individualized
result called a Breast Cancer Recurrence Score. My score came
back at 41. A 41 score falls into the High Recurrence category so

chemotherapy is helpful when determining my treatment choices.
I have decided to do my treatments at the University of California at
San Francisco Mt. Zion. I pick out my long blonde wig this Monday,
August 15 and plan to have my head shaved on Friday, August 26.
My doctor says hair falls out about 14 days after the first chemo
treatment. The kids start school on Monday, August 15. This is a big
day for my son as he is starting Kindergarten. I will be there taking
pictures. Thanks for all your good healing energy and prayers.
You are all very special to me.
Love,
Hillary

August 18, 2011

Chemo starts for me on Thursday, August 18 and runs every two
weeks for four months. After that time I have five weeks of radiation
from January 10 to February 23. Chemo dates are **September 1, 15
and 29 and then October 13 and 27, November 10 and 22**, first
with the chemotherapy drug called AC (Adriamycin) and
(Cyclophosphamide) followed by the chemotherapy drug called
Taxol.
Love,
Hillary

NOTE: As it turned out, I decided against taking the pharmaceutical
drug, Tamoxifen, after chemotherapy and radiation which was a
personal choice. I decided I wanted to steer towards a more natural
approach to control my estrogen and improve my health.

September 25, 2011

Hi and thanks ahead of time, my friends. Here's the schedule.

Monday, September 26 - Lafayette park with kids.

Tuesday, September 27 - Marina library and Moscone park with Randa after school.

Wednesday, September 28 - Cathy picks up the kids from school 1:50 pm - 3: 30 pm and I pick up the kids at Cathy's apt and bring them to Lafayette Park.

Thursday, September 29 - Chemo day. Mai Mai drives me to UCSF for an 11:30 am - 2:30 pm infusion. Heidi picks up Anna from school and brings her home at 5 pm. I know we do not have hip hop class so do what is best and Shadra picks up Tomas at 1:50 pm and brings him home at 5pm. My babysitter Margarita is going to try and be at our apartment by 4 pm on Thursday to cover so this means Shadra can drop the kids off closer to 4:30 pm if that works better. Julia, my son's Godmother flies in from Denver and should be at the apartment by 5 pm and is with us until Saturday morning.

Friday, September 30 - Merideth walks the kids to school and Julia picks them up at 1:50 pm and takes them on an outing. Rudi is home at 10:30 pm from Ottawa.

Saturday, October 1 - Margarita arrives at the apt 1 pm - 5 pm and takes kids to Lafayette Park.

Sunday, October 2 - Randa and Marie Jo take the kids to the park
1 pm - 4 pm and Rudi will drop them off and pick them up from your
apartment.

I am usually getting back on track on day 5 after chemo.

Thank you so much.
Love,
Hillary

October 19, 2011
Hi, I'm sorry it has taken me a while to respond but I have had a lot
going on at home with the kids and Rudi has been away traveling a
bit for business. I just finished my fifth round of chemo with three
more to go. Hurray!

Rudi had to be in Ottawa Canada for business for a week during the
September 29 infusion so Julia, my son's godmother, flew in from
Denver to be with me. Mai Mai was a total star and went to my
chemo Infusion with me. I thank them so much for being here.

Rudi was in San Diego on business for this new round of
chemotherapy called Taxol that I started last Thursday, October 13.
Fortunately, Cousin Betsy was in town from LA and she came to the
hospital with me along with Laura so I thank them very much for
sitting with me and for keeping me company. Margarita spent the
night and helped with the kids so I had good cover while Rudi was
away. After this last round of chemo on Thursday, I had a bad
reaction on my hands. They became red and swollen and were
painful but after taking Glutamine and having my hands inside
icepacks for a couple of days the swelling subsided. Strangely,
my big toes and heels of my feet were affected as well. Despite

everything going on, we had some fun this weekend with the School Halloween Carnival on Saturday which the kids loved. Anna went as a Swan Princess and Tomas dressed up as a dinosaur.

Anna helped me run the penny drop booth for Tomas' classroom which was a very popular booth. Sunday we went to Clancy's pumpkin patch which was very festive with lots of Halloween decorations and we picked out pumpkins to carve this Sunday. I wanted to thank you all for your ongoing support. I love you all. My next chemo infusion is October 27.
Love,
Hillary

October 15, 2011
To my friend, Jen P.

Thursday was a day, Jen. I was at the hospital for blood work at 8:30 am, followed by a cancer study meeting where I filled out cluster study questionnaire booklets, followed by 9 am - 12:30 pm ultrasound and three fine-needle aspiration biopsies on my right breast (mystery spots which were little cysts). The doctor had to insert tiny metal chips but they believe these spots to be benign cysts, followed by a follow-up doctor appointment and then a 3 1/2 hour Taxol chemotherapy infusion from 3 pm - 6:15 pm. So thank you so much, Jen, for being there for me and helping with food for the kids. I can't thank you enough. The Taxol has swollen my hands and fingers. At the moment they are red and dry and a bit tingly so that I can't bend my fingers well. I hope this subsides soon. I don't love this side effect. I only have a little tingling on my feet but mainly on both my big toes. This is very strange.
Love,
Hillary

PART II

ALTERNATIVE HORIZONS

Each moment is just what it is. It might be the only moment of our life; it might be the only strawberry we'll ever eat. We could get depressed about it, or we could finally appreciate it and delight in the preciousness of every single moment of our life.

- Pema Chodron

Chapter 4

DISCOVERING ACUPUNCTURE & MASSAGE

I was absolutely determined to regain my health. My thought was to throw everything at this cancer with both Western and Eastern medical practices. I was fortunate to have health insurance but the medical bills were still very high and many of my alternative treatments were out of pocket expenses. It's important to persevere, see the upsides, strive for positivity and make the best of an unfavorable situation. It's also very normal to feel pretty upset about a cancer diagnosis with deep sadness, anger and grief. You process it all and feel a wide range of emotions, the good, the bad and the ugly and hope for the best outcome.

The Alternative treatment which helped the most with my recovery was acupuncture, an ancient Chinese medical treatment that involves inserting thin needles into different areas of the body to help with "Chi", life force energy, relief from pain, various ailments and conditions as well as stress. The purpose is to bring your body back into balance.

It was through my friend Laurie that I found out about acupuncture. My oncologist put me in touch with her as I had asked to be introduced to another patient who lived nearby with the same breast cancer diagnosis as me. I wanted to find out what Laurie specifically did to support herself through symptoms. She was convinced that acupuncture really helped and she highly recommended her own acupuncturist to me.

Laurie and I met at a local restaurant near my apartment. It was comforting to know that there was someone else living nearby, with my same diagnosis and treatment plan who had successfully made it through treatment. I was a little nervous on my first Acupuncture visit as I did not know what to expect. My practitioner was called Jumbe and he had a heart full of compassion, a wise demeanor and a calming voice that immediately put me at ease. He explained how acupuncture would help me with my red and white blood cell counts, detoxification and building my immune system as well as easing symptoms of foggy brain, fatigue, constipation, nausea, mouth sores, dry mouth and neuropathy – pins-and-needles tingling sensation in the hands and feet.

He asked to see my tongue as he felt my pulse and I thought the whole experience was interesting. I lay on the table staring at the tapestry rug on the ceiling. Jumbe put acupuncture needles all over my body, between my eyes, on my hands and ears and on the top of my scalp. The needles did not hurt as they were quickly inserted. A heat lamp was placed near my legs. To my surprise, I found this whole process relaxing and meditative and I enjoyed listening to Jumbe's Zen stories and the calming music softly playing in the background.

On one of my visits, I asked Jumbe why he thought I got cancer. He said, "Hillary, you got cancer because you did." I love this answer. Jumbe explained why people might not think about or prioritize their health because many people are busy and distracted with day-to-day life activities; working, planning meals and eating, driving, spending time on computers, phones, social media, grocery shopping, washing dishes, doing housework, paying bills, watching TV, reading, going to the gym, outings with friends, caring for children, family and pets, attending or watching sporting events and focusing on various home activities and then repeating their routine over and over again every day like the movie Groundhog Day.

Jumbe's explanation made a lot of sense. I tried not to overthink this conversation in my mind but instead to still my mind and envision a glass of water. I fell asleep only to wake up 30 minutes later feeling completely refreshed and rested as if I had been asleep for a full eight hours. Here's the real significance: I actually felt fine after chemotherapy treatments with acupuncture. How could this be? I was curious about why and read the book in his office: *Between Heaven and Earth, a Guide to Chinese Medicine* by Harriet Beinfield and Efrem Korngold.

Massage work with Leslie

I started massage work just before my chemotherapy treatment phase to help relax and to cut through the anxiety I was feeling. I found a local Spa within walking distance from my apartment that offered Swedish massage and made an appointment with a massage practitioner named Leslie. As it turned out Leslie was not only an excellent massage therapist but also a true holistic empathic healer with a warm and caring personality and a great sense of humor. Over time and multiple sessions we became friends and spent time during massage talking about a variety of different subjects and life reflections.

Leslie had done her research on holistic wellness information and she was extremely knowledgeable. I learned how massage is restorative and works in a natural and healthy way to release tension from your body. Massage reduces cortisol which is produced by stress and helps with anxiety and your mind body and spirit. It releases and eliminates toxins, breaks down scar tissue and lessens pain in muscles while getting to the deep layers of fascia to increase mobility. Massage also improves blood circulation and boosts the immune system, assisting the body in the process of natural healing. After my massage sessions with Leslie, I always felt much better -

19

more relaxed, revived and happier as massage releases endorphins.

She also introduced me to a long list of holistic health studies and alternative therapies, from Dr. Masuro Emoto's work on the effect of human thought on water, the power of the Rife Machine, to the Akashic records and Bruce Lipton's book on epigenetics, *Biology of Beliefs*. I especially appreciated hearing about the inspirational story of Norman Cousins who cured himself of a degenerative disease through positive emotions and laughter. I also learned to avoid cancer-causing substances and additives such as artificial sweeteners and parabens, an endocrine disrupter that is a common ingredient in cosmetics.

Friendships with practitioners that develop through a cancer experience are often deep, comforting and meaningful relationships as they live through the healing process alongside you. Leslie had a great impact on my life and we kept in touch after she left San Francisco for West Palm Beach Florida. To this day I continue to get massage as part of my self-care regimen.

Chapter 5

THE HEALING POWER OF ENERGY WORK AND PRAYER

Be like the sky. The sky is always there, it doesn't complain.
It doesn't stop the clouds. You are in beingness – just let moods,
feelings emotions and thoughts float by.
Be in your silence and that will glow within you.

- Mooji

While going through chemotherapy, I contacted a good friend and classmate of mine from high school, Deirdre who is an energy healer and runs a holistic website called *Earth Clinic.* My friend encouraged me to make an appointment to see Bob in San Francisco for Reiki, hands-on energy work. She said, "Bob is one of the best energy healers in San Francisco, Hillary." I was curious. I had no idea what an energy healer even was at the time. So, I ordered a book online which I received for Christmas, *Wheels of Light Chakras, Auras and the Healing Energy of the Body* by Rosalyn Bruyere.

When I got up the courage to call Bob, I thought his voice was peaceful and soothing. My friend let me know Bob went to see John of God in Brazil many times during the year and I wondered—"Who is John of God?" I looked him up on YouTube and sure enough, John of God lives in Brazil and heals people from all over the world at the Casa Via touch healings, entities, and spiritual surgeries. Oprah Winfrey has been to the Casa and created a documentary on John of God's healing that I watched intently. Wayne Dyer also had a spiritual healing by John of God.

When I showed up to my first appointment with Bob, I was feeling fatigued, foggy-brained and anxious, common chemotherapy symptoms. During and after Reiki energy work I felt a sense of overall calm and well-being. By the session's end, my body felt warm and relaxed.

During one energy healing session with Bob, I learned about my Egyptian Astrology, my colors, my numerology and life path. I remember Bob asked me point blank if I was ready to pass on and I answered definitively, "No." I wanted to raise my children and I also wanted to travel the world. I wished to live and I knew in my heart I wanted to stay here on earth not only for myself but also for my husband, children, mother and my extended family and friends. I was going to be resilient and survive cancer.

I was introduced by Bob to John of God Casa Tour Leaders, Diana Rose and Bob Dinga, who travel together to Brazil several times a year to bring groups to visit John of God for healing. They presented my photo of me dressed in all white and placed a hand-written letter in the prayer basket at the casa and upon their return sent me blessed passionflower herbs in a supplement form that assisted with my individual healing.

I also read and listened to the work of an energy healer on one of my favorite websites called, MindBodyGreen, named Marci.

I gravitated to her articles explaining energy healing and listened to her five-minute meditations.

Marci is a Homeward Bound Guide specializing in energy clearing and transformation. She explains that Home means arriving at who you are, without labels, without the roles, without the stuff. It's the place where you finally land after searching outside. I learned that energy healers open themselves up as a channel to bring life force into the body and help trigger one's own healing system with the natural ability to self-heal.

Marci explained that energy healing releases blockages so you feel energetically lighter, calmer and happier. It clears stress and tension to allow for deep relaxation. One way that energy healing is supportive is that it acts as a conduit of universal energy and clears negative emotional, mental and unexpressed thought patterns that can get stuck in our body tissue. Energy healing accelerates the body's natural ability to heal itself and increases vitality.

Spirituality and Prayer

I was baptized Episcopalian. Growing up, I attended church on occasion with my father mainly on holidays. My mother's church was always in the garden. Spirituality for me is personal and private like many people feel about their faith. When your defenses are gone and you are left blown open and vulnerable with an illness, such as cancer, your thoughts may turn to the spiritual realm for hope, strength, courage and inner peace. My faith and spirituality were rekindled going through my cancer experience.

Prayer connects you to your inner soul, heart and spirit and to the divine. When faced with a life-threatening illness, prayer, whether individual prayer or collective, provides comfort, inner peace and emotional healing. Faith and prayer brought spiritual reconnection to my life. I prayed to a higher power to restore my health to wholeness and wellbeing. I prayed for myself and I blessed others. I read the book, *The Gentle Art of Blessing* by Pierre Pradervand for spiritual healing inspiration and to make a difference for myself and for others. I walked down the street in San Francisco and silently blessed others. I prayed on my hikes in nature or while lying in bed in contemplation. My friends and family let me know they were praying for me. Acquaintances and strangers I met let me know they would pray for my recovery. During diagnosis and treatment, I prayed for healing and recited The Lord's Prayer many times, the main and only prayer I've memorized since I was a child and can recite by heart.

Our Father, who art in heaven
hallowed be thy Name,
thy kingdom come,
thy will be done,
on earth as it is in heaven
Give us this day our daily bread
and forgive us our trespasses,
as we forgive those
who trespass against us.
And lead us not into temptation
but deliver us from evil.
for thine is the kingdom,
and the power, and the glory,
forever and ever. Amen.

One of my favorite spiritual teachers I found through the internet was Anita Moorjani. I became fascinated by her story and read her book while I was going through treatment, *Dying to be Me*. Anita's book is her awe-inspiring story of her Near Death Experience (NDE) from late end-stage cancer when she was in a coma, crossed to the other side, experienced the heavenly realm, discovered and understood who we really are, and then came back and recovered to full health to become an author, international speaker and spiritual teacher.

She taught me to listen to my inner voice and to understand we are more than our physical self. Through her NDE, Anita learned the bigger part of us is non-physical and the part that is nonphysical is far greater than our body. What is your purpose in life? Your soul, your consciousness has a reason for being here.

She teaches you to believe in yourself, to be aware and to proceed with confidence. If you believe in your ability you can manifest something in your life. Passion, love and joy are healing emotions. Don't judge yourself and instead observe yourself with no judgment. Anita confirmed, "We are all spiritual beings having a human experience." Her loving messages of self-love helped me during my most vulnerable time. Anita says, "Love yourself like your life depends on it; because it does." And she is right.

I realized I had to look deeply within myself, at my soul level and let go of fear to heal my Body, my Mind and my Spirit.

Mind and Meditation

Jasper is an icon in my neighborhood here in San Francisco. He has sat in the same spot for years at the bus stop outside of the Walgreens pharmacy on Polk Street often with his Street Sheet resting in his lap and recently two dogs at his side.

Soon after I was diagnosed with cancer he gave me a hug and said, "It will be okay, Hillary. Cancer is all in your mind." I appreciated hearing this from him as he has persevered through so much in his own personal life. Jasper's attitude has always made me smile. He is upbeat and friendly and remembers and calls everyone by their first name as they walk by him on the street. Our community rallies around him. He brings good cheer and wide smiles to passersby with his witty remarks and upbeat commentary. He is also thoughtful, saving me parking spaces, gifting me his sister's autobiography and watches owner's dogs while they are shopping inside Walgreens.

Jasper's remark about "cancer being in your mind" has stayed with me through the years. When I had a recent conversation with him about his comment he said, "Hillary, you don't even know you have cancer until the doctor tells you that you do. Your mind will help you recover from cancer. "

What I learned going through cancer is the mind is powerful and has the power to heal you. I paid a lot of attention to many thought leaders, and the work and mindfulness of Buddhist teachers, Pema Chodron and Thich Nhat Hanh. I also listened to my acupuncturist, Jumbe Allen. Jumbe explained how to breathe deeply from my diaphragm laying on my stomach and how to visualize healing light. I learned through Jumbe to turn my mind off and think and identify with "nothing," just focus on my breath, slowly breathing in and breathing out only. Counting sheep seemed easier. How do you go from a busy morning of multitasking and playdates with children to transition to thinking about "nothing" in acupuncture? This exercise required concentration and mindfulness. I would work at quieting my mind and focus on my breathing on my daily walk around the neighborhood or in bed before I fell asleep at night, in the middle of the night or in the early morning hour before starting my day.

While recovering from treatment I also started reading and watching videos of the work of Dr. Joe Dispenza. In his book, *Breaking the Habit of Being Yourself*, I learned that by tuning into the stillness of meditation you can change beliefs and perceptions. I listened to Joe explain how to rewire your brain and change your thoughts and beliefs. Here are some takeaways from his videos:

☐ Change your mind and change your life.

☐ The mind has a powerful influence over your physical self.

☐ The brain communicates with the body on a cellular level.

☐ Think differently, break your habits and you show up differently into your new self.

☐ You can't wait for your healing to feel wholeness. You have to feel wholeness to heal.

☐ If your brain and body have physically changed this is the moment to relax. The experience will find you and you will break the habit of your old self and live your new self.

☐ Lose your mind and create a new mind.

☐ Move from your old self to your new self.

☐ You have to feel empowered in order to feel success.

☐ You have to feel abundant before the abundance begins.

☐ Think greater than the conditions in your life and the environment to find freedom and joy.

☐ Focus on nothing, empty space - that is when the brain waves slow down but get highly organized and coherent.

☐ With meditation and being in the present moment, you become pure consciousness.

☐ If you change your thoughts and make new choices, you create new behaviors and new experiences and open to new emotions. Many illnesses are believed to be rooted in emotions and ideally can be cured by controlling these emotions. The brain is primed in its circuitry to not live in the past.

PART III

IS CANCER A GIFT?

Life is glorious, but life is also wretched. It is both.
Appreciating the gloriousness inspires us, encourages us,
cheers us up, gives us a bigger perspective, energizes us.
We feel connected. On the other hand, wretchedness--life's painful
aspect--softens us up considerably. Knowing pain is a very important
ingredient of being there for another person.

When you are feeling a lot of grief, you can look right into
somebody's eyes because you feel you haven't got anything to lose-
-you're just there. Gloriousness and wretchedness need each other.
One inspires us, the other softens us. They go together.

- Pema Chödrön, *Start Where You Are: A Guide to Compassionate Living*

Chapter 6

A GIFT AND NOT A GIFT

A friend of mine and I had a discussion about this paradoxical truth. How can cancer that is clearly not a gift also be a gift? Cancer treatment and recovery mean months on end of surgeries, chemotherapy, radiation, out of pocket alternative treatment followed by a period of intensive recovery time.

The experience of cancer can also be looked upon as a real growing time, filled with touching and deep tender moments. It is an accepted truth the hardest and most difficult things you go through in life sometimes provide the greatest opportunity to grow. The gift is being able to see the beauty through the muck. The gift and beauty of life are heightened for you when you are faced with the opposite – a disease. The duality of the situation you are in allows you to see the light vs. darkness on multiple levels.

From the viewpoint of treatment, chemotherapy also reflects a similar duality. Chemo is a gift in that it kills fast-growing cancer cells, and destructive because it also kills healthy normal cells. It's a long sitting process to receive the infusions and exhausting going through the symptoms post-chemotherapy. After chemotherapy treatments, I was fatigued and had foggy brain and did not remember who called me, what I said or what I did. My husband had to orchestrate all my anti-nausea medications because I was so foggy-brained. My taste buds were not the same after chemo and foods tasted bland and metallic. I was also not very hungry and my weight dropped significantly.

The gift was all the love, patience, support, cheerleading and generosity from friends and family, with calls, cards, help with children's schedules, rides to chemo infusions and green juices, soup and meals dropped off to our home from food delivery and friends. The support, love, encouragement and caring were essential for my recovery. I also learned people truly want to jump in to help others. Before cancer, I used to be more lopsided, feeling more comfortable giving than receiving, but one of the gifts I learned was how to receive with grace which in turn creates more balance.

Before starting chemotherapy I had an echocardiogram, Transthoracic Echo, to test the strength of my heart to endure the rounds of chemotherapy. I also shaved my hair off instead of watching it fall out which was a practical and humbling move of mine and brought control to an emotional time. My husband and friends, Laura and Jennifer who showed up to support me and bring cheer and kindness on my hair shaving day at a local hair salon was the gift. I bought long blonde wigs but they were uncomfortable and itched my bare scalp so I decided to wear hats instead which was not only a practical solution but far warmer and more comfortable. My aunt provided a cleaning service as a gift while I was going through treatment which was extremely helpful as my priorities were focused on getting better.

Combating Symptoms

After my initial chemotherapy treatment, I had bed-soaking hot flashes at night that soaked through the sheets to the mattress. The sheets would be so wet I had to get up in the night and change them. This was followed by the stoppage of my menstrual cycle after the first round of chemo never to return again. This was a life transition. I was surprised as I was not anticipating a sudden finality to my menstrual cycle at 45 years old. The first chemotherapy I was on was called AC - doxorubicin hydrochloride (Adriamycin) and

(Cyclophosphamide) nicknamed, "The Red Devil" due to side effects and its red color and challenging side effects. The effects of AC were cumulative. I had a vial of blood taken before every chemo to check I was okay to have chemotherapy. After chemotherapy, I had a Neulasta shot which increases white blood cells to decrease the chance of infection.

I lost a toenail with chemo and had a fingernail abscess drained from a painful infected nail while battling mouth sores, ongoing night sweats, a herpes outbreak, red and burning painful hands and feet with neuropathy – a feeling of pins and needles in my hands and feet. When preparing for radiation I was not expecting the lazar dot identification tattoos on my breast. I was not forewarned by the radiologist of the tattoos needed nor was I expecting unforeseen constipation. It is alarming and anxiety-provoking going through unpredictable treatment symptoms, and it's tricky to wrap your head around the gift at the time when you are struggling physically and emotionally, but I reminded myself that at the end of the day, the treatments were helping me to heal and to have patience with the process. I had great doctors, nurses and alternative practitioners behind me, encouraging me. I was doing the best I could to stay positive, constructive and in the moment. In times such as this when days sometimes feel pretty bleak, you find your core inner strength and resiliency and you learn who you really are. This is perhaps a rare gift that is given to you.

Other Perspectives
Cancer presents struggles, hurtles and sometimes scary experiences and it also gratefully offers silver linings. I was fortunate and blessed I had completed my family as I already had my two children born in 2004 and 2006 before I was diagnosed with cancer.

In 2003 at the age of 36, I was on vacation at a bed and breakfast in Calistoga California when I conceived my firstborn, my daughter, and I had no idea I was even pregnant for some time. Before getting pregnant with my daughter I had a miscarriage at six weeks, followed by polyp surgery, so I was not anticipating getting pregnant so quickly after the surgery. I put off going in to get tested to see if I was having a viable pregnancy as I was spotting every day and I didn't want to receive disappointing news.

However, when I finally got up the courage to go to my ultrasound appointment and looked at the monitor, I was blown away at the developing fetus on the screen. The ultrasound technician let me know I was almost three months pregnant and I cried with happiness. The best day of my life was seeing my daughter's face for the first time at my c-section. My beautiful son arrived 23 months later also by c-section. Experiencing birth and the unconditional love you feel for your newborn baby is one of life's extraordinary moments, a divine gift. Having children who were depending on me for their survival gave me the clear focus, determination and courage to prevail and heal from cancer.

Chapter 7

THE CHALLENGE OF SELF-CARE

How do you define 'taking care of yourself'? Create a new self-care practice today. Observe your comfort level when it comes to being good to yourself. Discomfort is a wise teacher.

- Caroline Myss and Peter Occhiogrosso

The gifts of cancer come in different forms—and learning how to care for myself was a big one that involved changing nearly every aspect of my lifestyle.

I Don't Have Time for Cancer

I had my sister-in-law Karin laughing one day when I said, "Where was I?" We were talking about where my mind had been before my cancer diagnosis and how things had shifted. An essential part of my healing process was learning that our beliefs are unconsciously shaped and they underlie our behavior toward ourselves, specifically affecting our self-care or lack of it. In order to create a new lifestyle pattern, I had to uncover and shift those beliefs consciously.

This kind of change is hard to make. If you haven't learned proper nutrition and self-care growing up from your family, then you will find yourself following the pattern of your family, though you may be unaware of it. You can't expect other people to teach you things that they haven't learned themselves. You remain in the dark until there is a wake-up call which in my case was cancer. Even if your friends coach you on wellness topics you won't accept their advice because you're not aware that your own unconscious beliefs are blocking the way.

Before my breast cancer diagnosis I was a 100% caregiver taking care of everyone else in my life with little thought to myself. When a friend once asked me who came first in my life, I readily admitted my husband and children's needs definitely came before my own.

I was catering to others and not focused on my own needs at all. I was going nonstop throughout my days concerned with my children, taking them to the park and activities, playdates, museums, organizing yard sales and free toy giveaways, making meals for our family and friends having babies, throwing baby showers, organizing parties and inviting friends and their children for dinner, often. I was not resting and recharging during the day or sleeping through the night because my children were waking up once or twice in the night and then getting up for the day at 6:00 am. I was always up with them in the mornings and never slept in past 6:30 am. I was pushing myself every day to keep up with a very fast pace on interrupted sleep.

I was dedicated to my children and I loved being a mother who created a supportive and nurturing home environment with fun-filled days but I was not taking very good care of my own needs. When I had the kids for extended periods when my husband traveled on business for two weeks or more, I would sometimes feel lonely, especially on the weekends, for adult company and conversation.

Before cancer, gumdrops were a snack and other than walking to the park I was not exercising. I used to say I was a soldier forging through the trenches. Overnight trips away with friends were non-existent. I was solely focused on taking care of my family during this time.

There is a psychological component to self-care. Many of us were raised to think we should put others and their needs before ourselves and that it's selfish to think of ourselves before others. We all know when we fly in a plane the flight attendants tell you to please put your oxygen mask on first before assisting others sitting next to you in an emergency. However, it gets complicated when as a mother, no matter how many children you have, and in my case a baby and toddler, often your nurturing instinct is to first and foremost take care of your children and prioritize them ahead of yourself and everyone else around you. But you can't help anyone else if you in your mind feel broken yourself. I was a full-time stay at home mother and self-care was not a part of or planned into my days. I realize some mothers juggle work as well as taking care of their children. Self-care needed to be built into my day through better time management with activities added to my electronic calendar blocking out time for walking, massage, acupuncture or just personal quiet time.

Realistically, if you have children, you have to figure out what you can afford financially for a babysitter, nanny or for daycare and whether family living close by are open and available to step in and help babysit so you can take some respite. Determining the correct balance for you and your family is unique to each family dynamic and continuously shifts and changes. Self-care and time management logistics are something you have to sit down with and think about carefully and then plan smartly into your daily schedule to keep you on track and accountable.

After the cancer diagnosis, things changed. The main change is that I woke up and decided I was going to make some lifestyle changes. I started taking control of my own health and researching wellness information. I studied everything from plant-based nutrition and massage to supplements and essential oils; visualization, meditation and acupuncture. I stopped putting so much emphasis on others and I diverted all that energy back to myself. I learned how to say "no" to an invitation and feel okay about it, especially if it was something that made me feel overextended or something that I honestly did not want to do. I started shifting old habits and patterns to my own self-preservation. I was also resting and sleeping more on the weekends, writing in my journal, reading and thinking of wellness topics and ideas for this book. I started seeing a holistic nutritionist and acupuncturist and I was exercising daily, even if at first it was just a brief 20-minute walk around the block.

I was fortunate to receive incredible support from friends and family both during and after my treatment. Even strangers gave me a hug. I received meals, emails, cards, prayers and gifts from people near and far. Next door neighbors dropped off green juices and friends stopped in to say hello, deliver homemade soup or a meal and help fold laundry, or just sit and talk with me. Friends whom I may have convinced myself did not care about me before my diagnosis I found out really did care. I realized how I was perceived by others and how I perceived myself. There was a real sense of clarity and self-acceptance and happiness that kicked in because I felt loved and supported. I found out that friends and family don't focus on what you look like from the outside, your true friends and family care about you from the inside and love runs deep. Not everyone receives this level of support going through cancer and I realize I was very fortunate to have people around me, caring and cheering for my recovery all the way.

Chapter 8

HEALING THE PAST

Pain is a pesky part of being human,
I've learned it feels like a stab wound to the heart,
something I wish we could all do without, in our lives here.
Pain is a sudden hurt that can't be escaped.
But then I have also learned that because of pain, I can feel
the beauty, tenderness, and freedom of healing.
Pain feels like a fast stab wound to the heart.
But then healing feels like the wind against your face
when you are spreading your wings and flying through the air!
We may not have wings growing out of our backs,
but healing is the closest thing that will give us
that wind against our faces.

- C. JoyBell C.

Cancer prompted me, as it does many people, to look at the past in a new light, from old romantic relationships and family dynamics to forgotten hurts and unprocessed grief I had not dealt with. From every chapter of my life, I saw new meaning. I reviewed decisions I'd made and I was able to see lessons in my experiences that I had completely missed.

As a result, I decided I wanted to live my life with more authenticity and meaning and show up differently in certain relationships. You work through old hurts and heartbreaks and realize their purpose and meaning in your life path was to teach you a lesson and learn something new about yourself. You may have completely missed the point at that time. Forgive yourself from your heart and then forgive others from your heart. You learn to forgive the past and come into the present. When you look closely at people's actions and try to put yourself in their shoes, it gives you the necessary perspective for what they may have been going through at the time. You realize why things didn't turn out the way you may have liked. You process it and then you—step-by-step—let it go.

Mother Relationship

I love my mother. My mother has a strong personality, a good sense of humor and is an organized task-driven woman. Growing up I was a pleaser and would follow her lead and direction. As a young girl, I would get up in the morning to find my mother's "duty list" waiting for me on the kitchen table, a list of chores that I had to complete after breakfast. In the spring, my family would open up our Rhode Island summer home that had been closed down for the winter. My friend and I were her spring cleaning team, responsible for everything from making beds, cleaning bathrooms and vacuuming to sweeping the cellar, to sponging off all the appliances, cutting back trees and shrubs to hauling brush outside in the yard. We even applied Cuprinol to the deck. What this taught me was a good work ethic.

Scoliosis

When I was a young teen from 1980 to 1983, I was diagnosed with scoliosis and had to wear a full torso Milwaukee back brace for three years. My mother took on the major role of helping me with my daily regimen of taking my brace on and off and driving me to hospital check-up appointments. This style brace had a white chin rest that extended from a front center bar with a silicon body mold that you had to open up from the back and slip around your torso. Two separate body mold pads hung from straps attached to the back parallel steel bars. These straps had to be positioned, adjusted and then strapped in tightly. My mother took charge to strap me into this brace twice daily, morning and night as I had to change my undershirt which I wore under the brace. I was allowed out of my brace for one hour a day to shower or play tennis or when the skin on my hip bone had become chaffed forming an abscess from the constant rubbing.

When I was a sophomore in high school my parents sent me to boarding school with my back brace. My roommate, Carolyn, would help me in and out of my brace daily. The brace was heavy, cumbersome and sometimes tight and uncomfortable. However, I did not complain as I had accepted this is just how it had to be and I understood it was temporary. I made the best of my situation. At the same time, I was wearing my brace, my skin broke out with acne on my face, arms and back. My dermatologist put me on oral Tetracycline and then suggested birth control pills to control my hormones from these breakouts.

What I learned through these experiences was sensitivity, empathy and compassion for others experiencing a disability or hardship and how to respond with understanding and thoughtfulness. Sometimes I would feel vulnerable and sad when I would get a hard stare or hurtful comment which made me feel awkward but I learned how to deal with all the stares and comments, persevere and take the high road. This experience and life lesson came full circle and helped me persevere through my cancer diagnosis, chemotherapy and radiation and stay grounded.

Sexual Inappropriateness
During this time of healing, I also confronted an inappropriate sexual experience that happened to me at 6 years old that I had denied for years. My parents were having a cocktail party in our living room in Rhode Island and one of the guests' teenage sons, who was

babysitting me in my bedroom, touched me sexually and threatened me, saying something bad would happen to me and my family if I told anyone. I kept the secret for years until I eventually told my mother when I was much older. My mother never went back to address the incident with the teenager's mother and I forgave her for not communicating with her friend.

Later, I learned through my cancer hospital cluster study that cancer patients may experience these emotionally charged sexual abuse experiences as young children that are brushed under the carpet and years later manifest physically in the body.

My Son Tomas

I also processed the time my newborn son was hospitalized with a very high fever. On February 4, 2006, just three weeks after he was born, Tomas woke up from his afternoon nap with a high 102.4 fever. In the emergency room, after a series of tests, doctors determined he had urinary reflux. I was then admitted with him into the hospital for three nights while he was on an IV, receiving antibiotics and going through tests. He had a grade 4 out of 5 reflux and 5 was the worst grade. This experience was internally stressful at the time even though outwardly I remained calm. I was pretty sleep-deprived as I was nursing him around the clock every few hours.

My Father's Death

When my father passed March 23, 2006, I did not cry or grieve his passing but held the sadness and suffering inside. I was in a daze with a newborn and a two year old. It took me a long time to acknowledge this grief, move towards it and give it a voice, but I finally did. What I've learned through cancer is that unprocessed emotional grief is not good for human health. You have to show up for your emotions. You have to cry and let the pain, suffering and feelings out. Suffering is part of life. It took me a long time to acknowledge grief, move towards it and give grief a voice.

As part of my healing process from cancer, I did a lot of self-reflection and cleaned out the internal closet figuring out what worked for me and what didn't. I reflected on my triggers and stressors, identifying them and my behavior and how I could manage future stressful reactions.

I came to appreciate my innate gifts and what comes naturally for me versus what I struggle with that goes against the grain. I focused on school and career choices and assessed the skills I learned and all the people I've met. I recognized my leadership skills and organizational skills. I processed my time living overseas in London during junior exchange in college and then moving to London again after I married my husband, Rudi, and what I learned through European experiences, work and travel.

PART IV

THE PEOPLE WHO CHANGE YOU

Love is the Frequency of Life, and Life is the Frequency of Love.

- Rumi

Chapter 9

FAMILY

I have always known that love, the people you love, family and friends and your pets, are the most important thing in life—but cancer brought it to the forefront and confirmed it for me. Trust in love here on earth and eternal love to get you through. Witness how the heart is deeply moved and touched. Trust that it will work out and open and listen to your heart.

When I met my husband Rudi at a trade show in Las Vegas, he walked out of the elevator door and into my life. It was love at first sight. After we spent three days together, I knew I was going to marry him. I just couldn't believe the soulful connection. You just can't explain this type of coincidental meeting with words—you can only feel it.

Going through breast cancer with Rudi showed me the gift of love. He was solid as a rock as he continued to support me and our kids, staying strong for the family in the darkest hour while I was just coping to get through each day. Rudi would say nice things to me, such as, "You look beautiful!" and "You are my special girl, I love you" even though I knew how I must look with no hair, no eyelashes or eyebrows. Additionally, my weight had dropped from 130 lbs to 110 lbs and I looked so thin and fragile. My children were really strong for me as well and hugged me, and would hold my hands in bed after storytime.

I remember going to my son's kindergarten classroom to read on story day while going through treatment and my son said to his class, "This is my Mom and she is bald." I was so touched I could barely get through reading the book without crying.

One day in February 2012, as I was just about to complete my radiation treatments, my husband's father, Rudi Sr., suddenly suffered a severe stroke and shortly after passed away while with his wife on a trip to Sydney, Australia. This was a huge shift in our family dynamics as Rudi Sr. was the patriarch of our family and we all loved and cherished him.

His death helped me realize all the wonderful things he has shown our family. He was family-oriented, heart-centered, warm, kind, affectionate and loving to both his family and friends. When I was out with him he was outgoing and charismatic even with people he had just met.

He would sit at our kitchen table quietly pondering many subjects. He had a great value system and deeply understood the important focus in life and how to treat people with thoughtfulness and consideration. He was very intelligent, inquisitive and had great patience. Before his retirement, he had worked 35 years as a high school teacher.

Rudi Sr. was the model of emotional support and unconditional love. He took our children to the local stationery store to buy holiday cards, then helped them create a message and get their cards out in the mail. He also engaged the children in cooking projects and took them out to the park or Crissy Fields. He put together a poster photo collage of them, a genealogy slide show, and wrote two books for us—an elaborate cookbook with photographs and a storybook about my daughter's favorite stuffed animal frog, "Froggy Friend."

My father in law was a minimalist with a non-materialistic focus and understood that "things" don't bring true happiness and you can't take your assets with you. He understood there is a difference between necessity and desire and how not to be obsessed with the materialistic aspects of life. He would say nice things to his wife, daughter, granddaughters and me calling us his "flowers of heaven." These moments confirm Rudi Sr.'s greatest gift of all – his teaching and impact on the power of love which has no bounds and is unchanging – the power of unconditional love.

Chapter 10

TEACHERS, FRIENDS AND NEIGHBORS

Each person holds so much power within themselves
that needs to be let out. Sometimes they just need a little nudge,
a little direction, a little support, a little coaching,
and the greatest things can happen.

- Pete Carroll

In this chapter I want to gratefully acknowledge some of the amazing
people who came into my life at this critical time.

Dorothy

Dorothy was a Master Life Coach, Spiritual Director and Minister
who taught at the Center of Excellence in San Francisco. In 1995,
Dorothy was the Minister at my close friend Cornelia's wedding at
Beaulieu Vineyards in Rutherford California where I was her Maid
of Honor.

Dorothy came back into my life when I was diagnosed with cancer
and gifted me a few counseling sessions. Dorothy and I often met
face to face or spoke over the phone. Our conversations revolved
around inner work, how I was feeling, working through family and
relationship dynamics current and past, talking through emotional
childhood feelings and experiences, clarifying spiritual beliefs and
discussing alternative health treatments.

Dorothy opened my mind to exploring elevated self-awareness
and perception, self-discovery and personal growth. She had me
thinking about becoming the person that could live the life

I deserved and experience more happiness, purpose and fulfillment. Dorothy had an empathic and loving heart and inspired people to serve at their highest potential and authenticity and to reach for their true self. I sent Dorothy an orchid and a special card after my counseling sessions ended. I will always hold her as a special woman in my life for her loving kindness.

Terry

Terry is a professional life coach and yoga coach who teaches contemplative inquiry, self-discovery and self-empowerment tools to heal. Terry helps set your energy toward authenticity, creativity and genuine love of self and others. She explains that self-love inspires the choice for love in all circumstances and with all humanity and self-love is the key to happiness and fulfillment.

Terry knew Dorothy and provided me with three-hour customized yoga lessons to increase my core strength and flexibility, and to support my healing.

Terry always read to me from her poetry book during our sessions together. I remember with fondness the beautiful poem *Wild Geese* by Mary Oliver that she recited. It meant so much to me because of its beauty and deep sensitivity. It's a blessing in life to know there are people in our world like Terry with so much compassion in their hearts dedicated to helping others.

Wild Geese by Mary Oliver
You do not have to be good.
You do not have to walk on your knees
For a hundred miles through the desert, repenting.
You only have to let the soft animal of your body
Love what it loves.
Tell me about your despair, yours, and I will tell you mine
Meanwhile the world goes on.
Meanwhile the sun and the clear pebbles of the rain
are moving across the landscapes
over the prairies and the deep trees,
the mountains and the rivers.
Meanwhile the wild geese, high in the clean blue air,
Are heading home again.
Whoever you are, no matter how lonely,
The world offers itself to your imagination,
Calls to you like the wild geese, harsh and exciting
Over and over announcing your place
In the family of things.

Cecilia

Cecilia was a Spanish bilingual kindergarten teacher who taught at my daughter's school and lived locally near Lafayette Park. She made such an impact on my recovery that I will share a story about our friendship. I used to see Cecilia out in the schoolyard and I took notice of her approach, warmth and dedication with the children. When the school year ended in June, I decided to recognize her kindness and dedication and bought her a gift certificate from Tully's coffee. Cecilia didn't know me too well at the time but appreciated the kind gesture and used the certificate to buy a coffee thermos. Later I found out she brought the thermos to school every morning for several years.

Neighborhood Hang-out

After school, each day my children and I used to walk up the hill from our apartment to our neighborhood park, Lafayette, a children's park with playground structures and also a dog park. We became close friends with a group of local San Francisco neighbors and their dogs and we would all meet and hang out in the same spot every afternoon to catch up on the day's news and throw balls for all the neighborhood dogs.

One afternoon in the fall, my children and I happened to spot Cecilia sitting on her own on the hill with her new dog, Maizy, a Jack Russell beagle. When we walked over to talk to Cecilia and pet her dog, Maizy and my kids instantly fell in love. Not only was Maizy adorable with her unique coat pattern but she was smart and full of energy and loved to play and fetch balls with my children.

After that, Cecilia started showing up regularly at the park with Maizy in the afternoons and we all got to know one another well in a short amount of time. We shared thoughts and reflections on teaching and children, holistic health and wellness, spiritual topics, travel, cooking, men and dating. I remember sharing with her how I met my husband unexpectedly when I was not looking and we both agreed, "If you are taking care of yourself, the universe takes care of you." Cecilia would often volunteer to bring my children with Maizy up to the park in the afternoons while I was recovering from a chemotherapy treatment.

During fall 2011, a single guy named Brian who also lived in the neighborhood started showing up regularly at the park to join us with his Golden Retriever, Harvey. Brian hung out near us but kept his distance while eyeing Cecilia from afar. Another dog owner friend, Michael, who was married to Peyton and had Jack, a German Shepherd and Lulu, a Swiss Mountain dog, found out he was interested in Cecilia and told Brian to ask Cecilia out on a date after her return trip from Chile. Brian followed his suggestion and in January 2012, Cecilia and Brian went out for dinner on their first date. They hit it off that very night and just two weeks later they moved in together. Brian lived close to our apartment so we would volunteer to take Maizy and Harvey out in the afternoons to the park as they both had become our surrogate dogs.

On September 14, 2013, my children and I attended Cecilia and Brian's wedding held at Lafayette Park. I looked after Maizy and Harvey during the ceremony. We have all stayed in close touch through several moves, job changes and the birth of their son, Max. The experience of meeting Cecilia remains a memorable time in my life; the supportive and loving community of friendships I made at Lafayette Park and the amazing dogs I met all helped in my healing process and recovery.

Ray

Ray was a friend I met at Lafayette Park who made a big impact on my healing process too. Ray was a dog lover and loved his boxer, Sadi, who was attached to his hip. He took wonderful care of her, taking her to work with him at Golden Gate Cycles. Every afternoon Ray would stop by Lafayette Park on a break from work so Sadi could wander aimlessly around the grass and he could have a chat with me and our dog adult friends. Ray would always say, "Kisses, Kisses" and Sadi would kiss my children on the face which they loved.

I saw Ray for a while every afternoon so he felt like family. When Ray held the SPCA event (he was out fishing that day but still held the event) at Golden Gate Cycles for the SPCA adoption open house and motorcycle sale, my children and I made the effort to attend. Not only was Ray caring but he was creative and clever. He wanted to find caring homes for dogs and cats and to show he's a thoughtful guy, handing out free hot dogs and waters to his friends and customers. That's the kind of person he was.

Ray always had a smile on his face and a story to tell and our mutual friend Peyton would always comment, "Ray is the best-dressed man in San Francisco. He has a nice cologne, too." We would all agree and he would have a huge grin on his face. I would greet Ray with a hug because he was warm and friendly and easy to talk to. I'd say to Peyton, "Ray is great with women because he is open to talking about all subjects." During our group conversations we spoke mostly about fishing, Ray's passion, all of us listening because he loved going on about where he found the most fish during his last fishing trip. Ray just loved it when he would hit the right spot on the Delta for the fish bonanza and his competition would be off to another location with no catches for the day. He had a sixth sense on where the fish were congregating and he knew the Delta well.

The most important thing for Ray was his family and he spoke highly of his wife, Liz and his children. I heard stories of how Ray and Liz met while house sitting, about Liz's accomplishment of making it to the Olympics for water polo and how he cherished her as a loving mother and wife. He spoke highly of his son Ryan's fishing feats and also complimented his daughter, Traci, and how much he really liked her new boyfriend she had recently met on New Year's eve whom she ended up marrying.

Ray was into fitness and the gym. He cared about health and we had lots of talks about his next chapter in life where he thought he might retire and open up an exercise and gym program for seniors. I had finished radiation treatment and he was always very fun to talk to, warm and caring which I appreciated very much. I had sent him a text that was never returned asking him if he wanted to contribute

to the fitness section of the Wellness Project. It came as a shock
for me and many of us at Lafayette Park when we heard of Ray's
sudden passing while on a fishing trip June 26, 2012, at age 60 from
an undiagnosed oversized heart. Ray lived what he taught; love for
family, friends and animals, follow your passion and enjoy life to the
fullest with all the precious moments in life because life is fragile and
can change in the blink of an eye.

Peyton

Peyton was Michael's wife and Mom to dogs Lulu and Jack from
Lafayette Park. She was older than Michael but young at heart and
fashionable, arriving at the park in her finest attire, leather jacket
and fancy shoes. She worked part-time for Saks Fifth Avenue,
Barneys and Nordstrom. As dressy as she might have appeared
most days at the park, she was also down to earth and a good sport
throwing balls for the dogs during a windy rain storm in her heavy
weather gear.

Peyton did not have any grandchildren of her own so she adopted
mine. She said to my children, "Call me your San Francisco
Grandma." She babysat my kids at my apartment or at her place and
my children adored her. She took them out for pizza and brought
cake to Lafayette Park on their birthdays. On my daughter's ninth
birthday, Peyton surprised her at her birthday party at the SPCA. We
all had a close bond. It was a very sad day for my family when we
found out Peyton had an aneurysm and passed November 15, 2015.
The world brings your heart to beauty and love mixed with passing
moments of pain, sadness and endings. We all loved Peyton and she
will be greatly missed.

Renee

Renee was a massage therapist I started seeing in 2009 at Mindful

Body Yoga Studio in San Francisco. She was easy to talk to and compassionate and she was an excellent massage practitioner and accomplished yoga instructor as she had trained in yoga under Jonny Kest. She also was very knowledgeable about holistic health and sincerely wished to help me with my back and scoliosis.

For a time I saw Renee for massage regularly and we became friends. On one of my visits to see her, Renee asked me if I would be interested in a part-time job at the yoga studio, making calls to her clients, and doing basic office work and light housekeeping. I appreciated her thinking of me because at this time I was not working and my children were both toddlers. I just couldn't figure out how I could fit in a job, even part-time, as I was still pretty sleep-deprived and full-on with the children's activities while my husband traveled on business.

About two years passed without me seeing Renee regularly. Life just takes off sometimes and sends people in different directions for a little while but as I was going through radiation treatment, I found out on one of my visits for yoga at Mindful Body that Renee had been out on leave with breast cancer treatment. So we reunited under different circumstances.

I found out one day Renee had volunteered to teach a yoga class at Mindful Body so I showed up to surprise her. Renee had come out of treatment and her hair was just starting to grow back but her energy was good and her attitude and zest for life was inspirational. After our group yoga session, I found out Renee's cancer had metastasized to her brain. This was devastating news to hear and process.

Shortly after the yoga session with her, we met at a restaurant in Cole Valley in San Francisco for lunch to discuss the Wellness Project.

I thought she might be interested in contributing information on the benefits of yoga. On another visit, I brought her soup to the Center for Peaceful Healing where she was living. We would sit in her kitchen and talk about feelings and emotions, dreams, ideas and observations on family, friendships, travel, holistic health and what it was like living with breast cancer. The basic day to day tasks for Renee were becoming increasingly challenging and she was documenting her cancer experience on video.

The last time I saw Renee my daughter and I delivered two containers of soup to her front door. She passed April 11, 2013, at age 32. Renee taught what she believed and brought to others: love, emotional support, gratitude, patience, kindness and hope.

Chapter 11

PEOPLE WHO INSPIRE YOU

Compassion is not a relationship between the healer
and the wounded. It's a relationship between equals.
Only when we know our own darkness well
can we be present with the darkness of others.

- Pema Chodrun

Some days are happy and some days are less than happy when
you have cancer. You can't spin your situation and feelings to
the positive and be happy all the time because it's not realistic.
However, I found people who have inspired me and shown a light on
my path, guides who helped me focus on gratitude and happiness in
times of need, remembering that happiness truly comes from within.

In October 2012, eight months after completing treatment, I traveled
with my friend Amy to the Wellness Conference in Pasadena to hear
Louise Hay and Dr. Wayne Dyer speak.

At the San Francisco airport, I passed some decorated Delta gates
with a halo of soft pink balloons along with breast cancer pink
ribbons attached to the counter with "Hope" signs. I asked the Delta
representative what was going on and she said it was "Breast Cancer
Awareness." I told her I was a breast cancer survivor and she told
me about Delta's pink breast cancer plane.

I took a picture of one of the pink balloons at the gates. The pilots
arrived wearing bright pink ties.

As I settled into the flight, my stewardess arrived with the drink cart and my cocktail napkin. On one side, the napkin said, "The Breast Cancer Research Fund – DELTA – Enjoy Minute Maid Pink lemonade." The other side read: "Taking Flight For The Fight Against Breast Cancer One Minute Maid Pink Lemonade At A Time." I smiled. I had recently learned sugar is not good for cancer so I chose sparkling water, sat back and enjoyed the flight to Pasadena.

Hay House Conference
Dr. Wayne Dyer gave the keynote address on Friday night. I love Wayne Dyer. He has so many wonderful, loving messages and his daughters are gifted. One daughter, Saje Dyer, got up in front of the audience and told a story about curing her flat warts at age 5 by talking to them and sending the warts love. "I love you and appreciate you but we can't be together anymore and you have to leave." She pictured them coming off her face and she manifested a clear result in three days. His other daughter, also super talented, sang a beautiful Whitney Houston song.

Wayne Dyer spoke of the recent course he had given in Maui on Divine Love. I always envisioned a father with an open personality like him, heartfelt and funny too. I laughed out loud at his jokes. On Saturday we heard Louise Hay and Cheryl Richardson. I didn't know who Cheryl Richardson was but my friend Amy knew her. Louise is now 86 years old and admitted her age but she seems so much younger. She discovered and was a major influencer in the self-awareness movement at age 45, writing the book that changed my life and many others, the famous *You Can Heal Your Life*.

Everyone hangs on to every word that Louise says. She is it. The Grandmother guru of self-help. Her hair is cut short now, she said, because she wanted "freedom from her rollers." I loved this statement. Louise and Sheryl were like two schoolgirls chatting on stage and I got the biggest kick out of their off-the-cuff banter, realness, and randomness. We began with some side hand tapping and this was fun. I had never done tapping before. The lights on the balcony level were too bright for Louise so she asked the stage crew to turn down them down and also to bring her a parasol. The next thing you see a parasol is being hand-delivered to Louise on stage and then a gentleman from the audience volunteered to come up and hold the parasol for her. This was funny and charming. I loved it. Here's what I learned from Louise:

- ☐ The first thing you say in the morning indicates how your day will be. Get up with a smile. Go to the mirror and say, "I love you." How you start your day is how your day is.

- ☐ You are an amazing problem solver. Don't focus on what isn't right. Say, "I bless and prosper everyone in the world and they bless and prosper me."

- ☐ Louise says bless all the appliances in your kitchen in the morning. Your kitchen is full of nourishment. Love and rejoice!

- ☐ Recognize and let go, which is a gentle process of learning.

- ☐ We want to love ourselves and not criticize ourselves. Be your best cheerleader always, be supportive of yourself and encourage yourself.

- ☐ Let me disappoint you. Saying "no" is okay. We are afraid of what other people think, that's how we create guilt and anxiety.

- ☐ Care less about what other people think.

- ☐ You are a radio station in your mind. Things can make you feel good or you can be upset. You are in charge of that dial. What can I think right now that would make me feel better? You are in control. You can go from unhappy to happy.

☐ You have the power to create the life you want – don't waste time talking about what you don't want.

Cheryl told a story I loved. She was in a restaurant handing out positive message self-help cards. She told the audience, "Fan them out and have your husband pick one and give one to the waitress. Don't stop there, pass one to the people sitting around you, too. Watch their reaction as they either relate to what they read or don't believe it but their friend confirms that in fact the message for them is true."

Another favorite author and speaker I saw in Pasadena is Robert Holden, whose book about happiness, *Shift Happens*, inspired me. He is warm, creative, funny, clever, and real.

Here are some of his powerful messages that I took to heart:

☐ There is more to life than the image we make of ourselves.

☐ Open yourself up to a deeper mystery.

☐ Unconditional self-love is self-acceptance.

☐ Wholeness and happiness are your true nature.

☐ Take a look at yourself. Who are you without your story?

☐ Uphold the memory of wholeness and come out trailing in glory!

☐ There is nothing wrong with us.

☐ The more you accept yourself, every area of your life improves.

☐ If you think there is something that is missing in your life it is probably you.

☐ The world is not just a physical place, it's a choice.

☐ Nothing makes you happy - your essence is already happy.

☐ We are here to follow our joy.

☐ The world has finished with your past if you have.

☐ Practice forgiveness – forgiveness is a miracle and sets you free.

☐ Grieve the past and come into the present tense.

☐ Your ego will never be ready to do your soul's work.

☐ It's never too late to connect with your heart.

Other wisdom that inspired me on my journey to healing came from authors Anita Moorjani, Eckhart Tolle, Emmanuel Dagher, Louise Hay, Mark Nepo, Mooji, Pema Chodron, Rick Hanson, Swami Rama, Thich Nhat Hanh, and Wayne Dyer.

PART V

THE LIFESTYLE OF PREVENTION

Optimum nutrition is the medicine of tomorrow.

- Dr. Linus Pauling

Chapter 12

MAKING LIFESTYLE CHANGES WITH CUSTOMIZED NUTRITION

Around the same time I was diagnosed with cancer in June 2011, my friend Jennifer who had been working on her own celiac disease convinced me I needed to make an appointment to see her functional medicine doctor, Dr. Sarah Kalomiros, a nutritionist, chiropractor and kinesiologist who practiced muscle testing and had put together a customized health and lifestyle nutrition program for her that she swore by.

At first, I was resistant. I could not see that I was doing anything different than anyone else around me. However, I had started being proactive with my health and I knew I had to make serious changes. Before being diagnosed, I had felt off for a while and was concerned about my low energy. I thought my fatigue was due to child-rearing and long periods of interrupted sleep with small children. It was around this time I read the book *Deep Medicine* by William B. Stewart, MD, which became a springboard for me to learn how to care for my health. A quote that influenced me, "Everything you think, feel, say and do is either health creating or health negating. Everything."

I went to see Dr. Sarah at least once a week while I was going through chemotherapy and radiation treatments and I learned a tremendous amount about nutrition and how you can support the body to heal through nutrition. The first day I filled out the intake form, which included a list of what I was eating daily and weekly: cookies, muffin mix, granola bars, gum drops, potato chips, etc.

What I was about to learn from Dr. Sarah was like going back to college. She explained most people are lacking the proper vitamins and nutrients in their regular diets due to over-processing and nutrient-deficient foods. The soil is depleted of minerals. She explained the importance of eating an organic plant-based whole foods diet with organic produce and plenty of cruciferous vegetables and keeping to pesticide-free and hormone-free food. Chicken should be free-range, grass fed, organic and beef grass-fed and sausages should say organic, no nitrates or nitrates added on the packaging while my eggs should not be exposed to pesticides, hormones and antibiotics as we take on anything the animal is eating.

Dr. Sarah taught me to be my best advocate and suggested that I remove refined carbohydrates, sugar, wheat and dairy from my diet since they are inflammatory and much of the wheat, corn and soy are genetically modified. She had me replace regular milk with almond milk and coconut milk and advised me to stop consuming soy because it mimics estrogen. She also recommended that I eat minimal portions of organic fruit such as bananas because of the high levels of sugar and she suggested blueberries and the berry family instead, for their antioxidants. She had me eating lots of nuts for snacking especially macadamia and brazil nuts as nuts are nutrient-dense and high in healthy fats as well as smoothies with coconut milk, spinach, half of a banana and frozen berries.

I added a whole avocado daily to my diet and ate so many sweet potatoes with organic chicken apple sausages to work at gaining weight. I ate wild salmon for Omega 3 and avoided swordfish and tuna because of the high mercury.

Along with my nutrition, Dr. Sarah added supplements and nutritional medical powder drinks. I was prescribed an extensive tailored supplement program. I would mix the nutritional medical powder with water and drink these 8-oz drinks three times daily at breakfast, lunch and dinner along with my regular meal. As my Oncologist was not sure how supplements interfered with chemotherapy treatments, I came off my supplements before chemo then resumed the supplement program five days after chemotherapy.

Dr. Sarah explained the nutrition program was like "sweeping up" after the chemotherapy treatments depleted me with deep cellular nutrition. I learned that one's body is very intelligent and has an amazing capacity to naturally self heal if treated and cared for properly with organic food and improved lifestyle choices. You can, with the right changes, recover from a serious illness like cancer and restore your health.

When I first started seeing Dr. Sarah I was inspired to bring back all of my old canned food to the local grocery store and received store credit. I used the credit to buy a white orchid for my living room. I rebuilt my pantry from scratch with healthier food choices and cooking oils such as organic olive oil, macadamia nut oil, walnut oil and avocado oil which does not turn food carcinogenic at high temperatures. She also asked me to buy the brand Aqua Panel water in glass bottles to avoid BPA. I followed her deep spring cleaning instructions.

I wanted to learn more about BPA. What actually is BPA, bisphenol A? The Environmental Working Group (EWG) in January 2012 sent around the following email:

BPA, a synthetic estrogen that can disrupt the endocrine system and has been linked to cancer, obesity, diabetes and early puberty, is allowed in food packaging. We know that BPA ends up in our children. The federal Centers for Disease Control and Prevention has found BPA in the bodies of nearly every person over the age of 6; EWG has detected BPA in 9 of 10 cord blood samples. Most canned foods are lined with a BPA-based epoxy that leaches into food and liquid in the can. EWG is working day in and day out to change the situation.

I learned to stay away from processed foods with dyes, preservatives, artificial flavors, high fructose corn syrup, partially hydrogenated soybean oil and refined sugar. They are empty calories. I now also watch for the Non-GMO labels (Genetically Modified Organism) at the grocery store as well as labels on cans that read "no BPA lining" as linings can leach into food and is an endocrine disrupter. I now buy Eden brand beans and Muir Glenn tomato products with BPA-free lining.

I learned that everyone has cancer cells in their body and if you have a healthy immune system you can fight it off. A strong immune system can destroy cancer cells. A whole foods plant-based diet helps build a stronger immune system, helps with sleep, hormonal regulation, blood sugar regulation and increases energy levels and mental clarity. Refined sugar breaks the immune system. Dr. Sarah explained sugar fuels cancer cells—it's like pouring lighter fluid on fire so I ate very, very minimal amounts of refined sugar. My change in food choices and my new whole foods cooking lifestyle suited me well, along with the added supplements, minerals, herbs and medical drinks. I started to gain weight and feel better and stronger and my energy became more balanced throughout the day.

After Chemotherapy: Infrared Sauna Detox and Coffee Colonic
After chemotherapy ended in November 2011, I began a series of

detox treatments sitting in Dr. Sarah's infrared saunas to eliminate all the toxins from chemotherapy. The intense heat from infrared saunas allowed me to sweat from every pore while strengthening my immune system and oxygenating cells. I remember sitting in this infrared sauna for as long as I could endure the intense heat, which was about 30 minutes.

I drank water continuously throughout the session as the sweat was beading up and pouring out of me. I periodically opened the sauna door for some relief and I could visibly see the chemotherapy seeping out from underneath my fingernails and I wiped this liquid away with a hand towel before entering the shower area to rinse off. These detox treatments relaxed and refreshed me and turned out to be an important post-treatment weekly routine.

I also followed Dr. Sarah's recommendation to cleanse my colon, using the "do it yourself" S.A. Wilson's organic coffee colonic enema kit purchased on the Internet. I followed the instruction manual and made the coffee mixture in a pot in the kitchen then brought the liquid in the enema bucket into the bathroom. The bucket of water and coffee mix hung from my shower head. A small long silicone tube ran from the bucket down into my hand as I lay in the bathtub. I put the end of the tube into my rectum and pinched the hose to control the amount of liquid flushing into my colon. I had to hold it in as I lay in the bathtub. Was I even doing this procedure correctly? I read the manual from the bathtub. This detox procedure was a bit awkward and I hoped it was beneficial.

Supplements

Dr. Sarah designed and personalized a program of supplements for my unique nutrition requirements, using kinesiology muscle testing. For prevention, I continue on many of the same supplements today that helped me get my health back on track during cancer treatment. You can research the benefits and also work with a nutritionist who is able to put together a tailored supplement program specific for your unique needs.

For more information on supplements, refer to The Wellness Seed Resource Checklist (page 136).

Chapter 13

RISKS AND ROOTS

Should you shield the canyons from the windstorms
You would never see the true beauty of their carvings.

- Elisabeth Kubler-Ross

How can the rug be pulled out from under your feet with an estrogen-positive breast cancer diagnosis and you didn't see it coming? Breast cancer statistics reveal that 1 in 8 women will be afflicted with breast cancer in their lifetime. Some authorities and researchers consider it a burgeoning epidemic. The question is: If you are not in the 5% to 10% women with genetic hereditary component, then how and why do you get breast cancer?

Statistics and Hearsay

Listed below are some of the risk factors that I'm aware of. These are stats and "facts" that have found their way into my brain after pouring through hundreds of websites and books. I don't claim to be current on the barrage of new studies and information released frequently. Some of the books listed in my resource section can address more medically researched and detailed facts.

- Exposure to chemicals and toxins.
- Depletion of nutrients, vitamins, and minerals.
- Breakdown of the immune system.
- Obesity and childlessness.
- High dose of oral contraceptives. I was on a high estrogen birth control pill from age 16 to age 32.

67

- 5% - 10% of breast cancer is hereditary, meaning genetic mutations passed from parent to child - BRCA1 and BRCA2 genes. Side by Side Sutter Health/CPMC fall 2013 study says only about one in 400 people carry the BRCA gene but it can increase your breast cancer risk to 80 percent.
- Girls having their period early in life before age 12 and being exposed to high levels of estrogen and women having children late in life and who go through menopause after age 55. I was age 12 when I got my period.
- Caucasian women have a higher risk for breast cancer, while African American women tend to develop more aggressive cancers. (Info from Side by Side Sutter Health/CPMC fall 2013)
- Dense breast tissue, high hormone levels and high dose radiation to the chest. I had torso radiation several times a year for scoliosis screening throughout my teens.
- Drinking alcohol raises the risk of some cancers.
- Stress as a catalyst.
- Cancer is a Perfect Storm!

How can you stay away from chemicals and toxins in the environment, food, water, pesticides in soil, and air pollution?

I learned about the Environmental Working Group (www.ewg.org) and their Skin Deep Database from my friend, Laura. I looked up all my beauty products and ingredients - soap, creams, sunscreen, sex lubricants, shampoo, toothpaste, hand soap and body wash, perfume, home cleaning products, laundry detergent, hand sanitizer and ended up replacing many with new brands with clean ingredients.

I threw away beauty products containing methyl and propyl parabens linked to breast cancer. I read on the Breast Cancer Action website (www.bcaction.org) in October 2013 that about 200 of the over 80,000 chemicals in use in the United States have been tested for human safety. One of my cousins had also told me about the Center for Environmental Health (www.ceh.org) that protects us from toxic chemicals in air, water, food and in products. I just read from the local hospital that parabens have some estrogenic action that is now starting to show some association with breast cancer.

Why aren't Americans being protected?
Dr. Taylor, MD, from Yale University said, "BPA looks like estrogen. It mimics estrogen while phthalates block testosterone action. The chemical stimulates uterine growth and animal studies have found genetic abnormalities in eggs and increased risk of mammary cancers. A 1998 study in the journal Environmental Health Perspectives shared that BPA stimulates the action of estrogen in human breast cancer cells."

Alcohol is a factor in breast cancer and cancer reoccurrence.
My Oncologist let me know that there may be a link between alcohol and breast cancer. Women who have had breast cancer are advised to drink two glasses of red wine a week tops - or none - to prevent against reoccurrence. Now, that's an eye-opener. The American Cancer Society says alcohol intake can also increase levels of estrogen in the blood. Esther Blum, MS, MD, said "Too much alcohol is toxic. The reason you feel lousy after a night's drinking is a combination of dehydration, hormonal changes induced by alcohol, the direct toxic effects of alcohol and inflammation caused by metabolizing alcohol, or the impurities in the beverage. When you drink your body converts alcohol into toxic byproducts that can cause free radical damage to the liver. This can impair your body's ability to detoxify itself."

I put together a straight forward **Basic Self-Care Regimen:**

Mind – Care for your mental state. Practice Meditation - lower your stress.

Social – Nurture relationships with others.

Emotional – Love Yourself, take care of yourself, meet your own needs, see a life coach or counselor to heal wounds.

Nutrition – Eating well is a form of self-respect. Look at a plant-based whole foods diet and cut out processed foods. Add more greens to your meals, juicing and tailored supplements.

Spiritual Care – Take care of your soul and spiritual health – Connect with a higher power through prayer, quiet time, join a community of like-minded others, walk in nature.

Sleep – Sleep 8 hours at night. The Breast Cancer website (breastcancer.org) states that sleep deprivation can cause low-grade inflammation which is linked to almost all types of cancer and heart disease. Dr. Eliaz says, "8 hours of sleep at night contributes to healthy cellular activity." Sleep is good for your immune system. During sleep there is repair work that goes on both keeping cortisol stress hormone in balance and also low cortisol is better for immune health.

Exercise – Walking and exercise is good prevention medicine. I read recently that sitting is the new smoking. Walk and move 30 minutes to 1 hour a day 6 days a week. Exercise oxygenates your blood and cancer hates oxygenated blood, regulates your hormones, protects your cell walls, builds your immune system, works on your lymphatic system, detoxifies toxins, cuts the fight or flight stress hormone cortisol, improves mood, keeps your muscles in shape, helps maintain healthy weight to name a few. Dr. Eliaz says, "Exercise helps you actively fight abnormal cell growth."

Chapter 14
WELLNESS AND MINDSET TIPS AFTER CANCER

You gain strength, courage, and confidence by every experience
in which you really stop to look fear in the face.
You must do the thing which you think you cannot do.

- Eleanor Roosevelt

Completing cancer treatment brought with it a strange feeling. I was happy to be on the other side of treatment and there was a sigh of relief but the transition was challenging. I discovered that I needed time to process what had just happened to me. Life continues and you begin again in the moment. The people who supported and circled around you while going through treatment go back to their day-to-day. You feel like a new version of your old self.

Cancer changes your perspective on life and changes your views on everything from family, spirituality, work and the future. Now I just had to dust myself off, keep smiling and keep going. Many people offer different ways to cope after treatment is over. A few important takeaways for me were simple. Be thankful. Enjoy each day. Spend quality and quantity time with the people and pets that mean something to you and focus on things you love to do. Out of a cancer experience I discovered comes ones deepest strengths, abilities and values. I was eager to get to work on writing the Wellness Project and share with others what I had learned about the healing process.

Taking responsibility for my health
When I started taking responsibility for my own health alongside my

western protocol of chemotherapy and radiation, it gave me hope and inspiration. I realized the person who is actually responsible for my health was in fact me. I researched and educated myself on alternative and holistic Eastern practices, talked to survivors, read holistic health books and nutrition articles, explored websites and watched endless videos while journaling through it all. As I accumulated this eye-opening knowledge and guidance, I realized that my extensive collection of wellness information would be beneficial for others.

Take a look at the wellness and mindset tips I've listed below. You can check the boxes of the ones you're attracted to, look into them further and give them a try. For more in-depth information, see the Wellness Resource Checklist.

WELLNESS TIPS

☐ Move to a whole foods plant-based diet and eliminate processed foods.

☐ Drink green tea throughout the day with lemon, lime, or fresh ginger for its anti-inflammatory benefits. You may not want to drink on an empty stomach.

☐ Drink filtered water from glass containers.

☐ Avoid storing your leftovers in plastic and use glass because research has shown that the BPA (Bisphenol-A) in plastic is an endocrine disrupter.

☐ Avoid refined sugar & carbohydrates (anything white) – sugar fuels cancer cells.

☐ Steer away from heating food in the microwave because it affects the vitamins and nutrients. Never heat plastic in a microwave.

☐ Eat more organic vegetables and fruit, 70% cruciferous vegetables (broccoli, kale, cauliflower, Brussel sprouts) and fruits such as blueberries, strawberries, blackberries.

☐ Buy your veggies and fruits from a local Farmers Market.

☐ Buy a Breville, Huron, NutriBullet, or Vitamix blender / juicer and make a point to drink fresh green juice every day.

☐ Eat a teaspoon of organic coconut oil every day.

☐ Look at your cooking oils and switch to organic. For example, organic cold pressed virgin olive oil, organic coconut oil, macadamia nut oil and avocado oil.

☐ Drink organic bone broth for vitamins and minerals and immune system support.

☐ Take turmeric supplements or cook with turmeric which is anti-inflammatory.

☐ Consult a Functional doctor or Holistic nutritionist who will tailor the best whole foods diet for you with added supplements to support your individual needs.

☐ Take Supplement Vitamin D3.

☐ Sit or walk in the sun without sunscreen for 15 minutes to get your natural vitamin D to enhance mood and energy through the release of endorphins.

☐ Take a teaspoon of apple cider vinegar every day to detox and raise pH.

☐ Walk to build your immune system, help lymphatic system, oxygenate the blood and circulatory system, protect cell walls, regulate hormones, and reduce cortisol levels.

☐ Exercise. Try intermittent exercise on a stationary bike (30 seconds of full out exercise then 90 seconds of slower speed).

☐ Avoid using skincare products with harsh or toxic chemicals. Consult database of products at ewg.org.

☐ Buy green laundry detergent and dish soap such as Ecover and Seventh Generation.

☐ Replace non-stick frying pans and non-stick cooking pots with stainless steel, cast iron, good quality enamel because chemicals leak into food.

☐ Wash hands after touching receipts as many receipts often contain BPA.

☐ Sleep 7 to 8 hours per night, ideally 10 pm-6 am. Deep sleep heals on a cellular level.

☐ Sleep helpers: black eye mask, black out shades, dark curtains, ear plugs, cbd tincture or gummies, warm bath with dead sea salts, melatonin, Ylang Ylang and Lavender essential oil, deep breathing, no alcohol, no caffeine in the afternoon, sound machine, reading before bed and no electronics including cell phones on your bedside table, turn WiFi off.

☐ Bathe with Dead Sea salt minerals to help with sleep, build the immune system, increase circulation, help skin, release toxins and provide magnesium, potassium, calcium, chloride and bromide minerals.

☐ Try Dry brushing – helps with detoxification, blood circulation and skin.

☐ Start a journal and write down what you are grateful for and how you are feeling.

☐ Read a book you love.

☐ Say Positive Affirmations and Mantras.

☐ Allow yourself relaxation and quiet time.

☐ Spend time with the people and pets you love.

☐ Listen to relaxing music. Pandora App, free meditative music, Native American flute music, and binaural beats on YouTube.

☐ Listen to *Getting Into The Vortex* guided meditation by Esther and Jerry Hicks.

☐ Rebounding. Jump on a mini trampoline to stimulate your lymphatic system.

☐ Boost your overall well being with massage: helps immune system, circulatory system, lymphatic system. It also reduces stress and anxiety, calms your mind, increases energy and detox, prevents stiffness, tones and rebuilds tissue.

☐ Stand on a vibration plate to improve muscle strength, bone density, and lose body fat.

☐ Visit a dentist regularly. Make sure you have root canals pulled as leaving dead teeth in your mouth can be toxic and have an implant inserted instead. Switch out mercury fillings to a safer material recommended by your functional dentist.

☐ Create and nurture a strong social support network.

☐ Keep laughing. Norman Cousins cured himself of a life-threatening degenerative disease through laughter.

☐ Practice yoga for stretching, core strength, sculpting, immune system, mind, body, spirit.

☐ Practice Meditation to help alleviate anxiety, come out of your ego. Connect with your true being.

☐ Practice breath work and prana exercises for proper breathing from your diaphragm.

☐ Get acupuncture to help your immune system, white and red blood count, put your mind at ease and detox.

☐ Consult a Reiki Energy healing practitioner. We are all energy beings.

☐ See a Life Coach, Counselor or Psychologist and heal emotional wounds.

☐ Practice creativity: drawing, writing, painting, crafts, expressive arts - calms anxiety.

☐ Use thermography to check breasts. Measures heat and detects at a cellular level and is nontoxic.

☐ Use infrared sauna to help detox at the cellular level, improve circulation, oxygenate the body's cells, strengthen the immune system, provide pain relief, and lower blood pressure.

☐ Sit in a steam room or sauna to detox.

MINDSET TIPS

☐ Love and value yourself.

☐ Take care of yourself.

☐ Love your friends and family unconditionally.

☐ Give and receive compliments.

☐ Create a support group.

☐ Love and nurture your pets.

☐ Find your inner strength.

☐ Focus on your resilience.

☐ Think positively.

☐ Work at correcting bad habits.

☐ Take charge of your life.

☐ Speak up and have a voice.

☐ Self advocate for your own self.

☐ Say repetitive "I am" positive affirmations.

☐ Speak your truth.

☐ Give encouraging words of support.

☐ Be a spokesperson and supporter for what is right.

☐ Focus on the greater good.

☐ Visualize health.

☐ Slow down in your day.

☐ Set goals for yourself.

- ☐ Take risks.
- ☐ Don't be attached to the outcome.
- ☐ Practice time management.
- ☐ Express your own individual authenticity with confidence.
- ☐ Practice forgiveness through your words and your actions.
- ☐ Concentrate on what is nourishing.
- ☐ Stay in tune with your body.
- ☐ Walk with a friend.
- ☐ Engage in life.
- ☐ Empower yourself.
- ☐ Set boundaries.
- ☐ Get inspired.
- ☐ Smile at people.
- ☐ Open your heart to the community.
- ☐ See and express gratitude in your day.
- ☐ Keep a journal of thoughts, reflections, gratitude.
- ☐ Write out your sorrow & express your grief.
- ☐ Have the courage to walk your own path.
- ☐ Become the person you want to be.
- ☐ Let go of your limiting beliefs.
- ☐ Remember that abundance is every human being's birthright.
- ☐ Keep hope alive.
- ☐ Time heals us.

- ☐ Become resourceful.

- ☐ Embrace change.

- ☐ Bring spiritual consciousness into your life.

- ☐ Create peace inside yourself.

- ☐ Focus on who you really are.

- ☐ Act with honesty and integrity.

- ☐ Envision a peaceful world.

- ☐ We are strongest when we are in our own power.

- ☐ Put intention into your daily activities.

- ☐ Send people thank you letters in the mail to express gratitude.

- ☐ Forgive yourself and others.

- ☐ Rejoice in the uniqueness of each person.

- ☐ Take responsibility for your own happiness, thoughts, emotions, actions.

- ☐ Remember that all things are possible.

- ☐ Realize the oneness in the world.

- ☐ Take care of the planet.

- ☐ Create transformation.

- ☐ Take time to laugh.

- ☐ Remember your spirit is free.

- ☐ Sing and dance.

- ☐ Travel to new places.

- ☐ Help others brings you happiness.

- ☐ Sit in silence.

- ☐ Breathe.

- ☐ Let go.

- ☐ Let your resistance go.

- ☐ Move forward with confidence.

- ☐ Raise your vibration.

- ☐ Create a sacred space.

- ☐ Say healing prayers.

- ☐ Simplify life.

- ☐ Declutter your home.

- ☐ Create meaning in your life.

- ☐ Surrender to the unknown.

- ☐ Trust in yourself.

- ☐ Treat yourself.

- ☐ Be generous to others.

- ☐ Connect with your inner self.

- ☐ Believe in your psychic abilities.

- ☐ Listen to your intuition.

- ☐ Reflect on all the things that bring you joy.

- ☐ Feel tenderness.

- ☐ Study the meaning of the word Grace.

- ☐ Pray for grace.

- ☐ Treasure your memories.

☐ Take steps to move from fear to love.

☐ Open your heart.

☐ Design your life.

☐ Cherish each moment.

☐ Have a purpose in life.

☐ Follow your passion.

☐ Gently move into your pain and suffering.

☐ Practice detachment.

☐ Practice empathy and compassion towards yourself and others around you.

☐ Detach from the outcome.

☐ Wait for the right timing.

☐ Help make the world a better place.

☐ Work on a hobby or project that brings out your best self.

☐ Surround yourself in nature.

☐ Practice grounding.

☐ Trees are very healing and bring oxygen.

☐ Accept the now and don't regret the past.

☐ Hold a vision and focus.

☐ Release old beliefs that don't suit you anymore.

☐ Dream big.

☐ Never give up.

☐ Recognize your divine nature.

☐ Reach for your higher self.

☐ Manifest your full potential.

Life is delicate and fragile – while you have the opportunity, create your purpose and discover what your path in life is. Focus on wellness and make the best of your time here on earth.

PART VI

CANCER STORIES

I am not what happened to me. I am what I choose to become.

- Carl Jung

This book started out as a desire to tell my story and share my healing process. Along the way, I met and made some amazing friendships with women who were also going through cancer treatment and who became critical to my recovery—so I decided to share some of their stories.

Everyone's cancer journey is a personal journey, each one making their own health and medical treatment choices. In the same way, some of my friends were open and communicative while others were private. There are many unique, deep and meaningful alternative healing routes represented here. I hope their stories broaden your perspective.

Gail

Gail came into my life on a Saturday at a cancer retreat held at the local hospital post-treatment in the spring of 2012. She had been diagnosed with Stage 4 breast cancer. We randomly selected to sit next to one another during a cancer retreat and I remember thinking, "Here is a woman of strength, character and intelligence."

Brook, the meditation teacher who was calm and lovely, took us through a guided imagery healing session and Barbara Musser, who wrote the book *Sexy After Cancer,* spoke on healthy sexuality and intimacy post-diagnosis. Standing tall, Gail spoke articulately about her views on mind, body and spirit, namely that the human spirit can endure a lot through grounded faith. I appreciated her sensitivity and candidness and gravitated towards her warmth and sincerity.

Gail and I became fast friends and now more than five years later, are still close friends. We have shared intimate conversations over lunch and email, struggles and accomplishments, wellness articles, religious topics, books on health and wellness, family stories, family photos and humor. Our discussions on alternative cancer subjects have bonded our friendship as soul sisters.

Silvina

Silvina was diagnosed with Stage 4 colon cancer at the same I was going through treatment for breast cancer. We met during a parent coffee school orientation, as her daughter was in the same first-grade classroom as my son. Originally from Uruguay, Silvina stood out in the crowd because she was beautiful and had a nice smile and a fun, upbeat and warm personality. She joked and laughed with all the school parents sitting around the conference table and it was apparent she had high emotional intelligence. Silvina was a dedicated mom, wife and daughter and loved and cherished her two children, husband and family. We would get together in the mornings after school drop off and discuss treatment results and nutrition ideas. I would bring over a meal and we would chat about living with cancer, how things were going in the moment, our feelings, fears and deep meaningful subjects.

After she moved away from the city, we stayed in touch for support. She was courageous and an inspiration to many through her ongoing surgeries, chemotherapy and radiation enduring treatments over the course of 5 years. She fought on to live as long as she could with the progression of her cancer to her bones and lungs. Silvina passed peacefully on February 12, 2017, at the age of 41 leaving behind a beautiful family, two young children and a large community of friends who love her dearly. You can watch her Vimeo slideshow and read her story on Caring Bridge under Silvina Nieves Meshel.

Lucy

Lucy was diagnosed with breast cancer at the same time I was diagnosed in June 2011. I met her at the hospital during her last week of radiation treatment. We got talking to one another outside the changing room and exchanged numbers. She was 39 at that time and had three young children, ages 2, 5 and 7. Initially, doctors thought she was stage 1 but after surgery it was discovered she was, in fact, stage 3 with extensive lymph node involvement. She went through a double mastectomy.

Lucy followed the full western protocol of treatment which consisted of five months of chemotherapy, six weeks of radiation and six years and counting of hormone suppressing therapy. She also did monthly shots to suppress her ovaries and eventually had an oophorectomy to remove her ovaries. During cancer treatment, she implemented many holistic practices including acupuncture and reiki, both of which helped her mitigate the harsh side effects of chemotherapy and radiation. At the same time she cleaned out all the plastic and nonstick pans from her kitchen and replaced toxic beauty products in the medicine cabinet. She also cut back on drinking wine and eating refined sugar, dairy and started juicing.

Lucy would come over to my apartment for lunch when she had her monthly check-ups at the hospital and we would exchange alternative wellness ideas and provide each other encouragement and support. We love recounting the time when we ran into one another unexpectedly on the street in Oakland when I was looking for a parking spot. We said to each other that we were fated to meet.

Lucy says the biggest change that came with cancer was her change in perspective. Today she strives to live in the moment and not let the little things in life get to her like she did before diagnosed, which she readily admits is easier said than done. She was extremely appreciative of the community that rallied around her during what she said was a gut-wrenching difficult time both emotionally and physically. At Lucy's five-year cancer-free milestone, she decided to get a small bird tattoo on her wrist. She says the bird symbolizes freedom, freedom from treatments and freedom from cancer, a huge milestone she accomplished in her life.

My Tahoe Friend

A friend and neighbor I met during my 2010 summer vacation in Tahoe, who chose not to give her name, was open to sharing her breast cancer story.

One day in 1998, she found the tumor in the shower and immediately made an appointment to get a mammogram. At first, her doctor did not think the tumor was cancer and sent her home but after seven months it had grown in size so she made an appointment at Stanford Medical Center where they discovered the tumor was, in fact, stage 4 cancer.

My friend explained how she went through surgery, six months of chemotherapy and three months of radiation. During what she said was a pretty hellish time, her husband and then 23-year-old daughter were not very helpful and she decided not to tell her friends.

Throughout treatment, she searched out many alternative modalities including traditional Tibetan medicine, traditional Chinese medicine, supplements, acupuncture and praying to different Native American tribes. Her grandmother and aunts had both been diagnosed with breast cancer so she knew she was at high-risk for a similar diagnosis. Before cancer she said she was more extroverted but after cancer became more reclusive and selective, choosing to reign in all her energy for her own self-protection, self-preservation and self-healing. Now, after all the time that has gone by, she has moved on and feels at peace with the end of the breast cancer chapter in her life.

Christine and Alexia
I met Christine and her daughter, Alexia, in the infusion room at the hospital. Christine happened to be on the same infusion schedule as me and we often sat near each other during infusions. They were both warm, friendly and conversational and I loved watching their mother-daughter connection and bond as they sat together quietly speaking French.

We all became friends going through this experience together and have kept in touch meeting for lunch, sharing in the joy of the birth of Alexia's son while corresponding on email which Christine always writes in both French and English.

Christine wrote:
Just after the end of a tough teaching school year in June 2001 and also while dealing with the painful possible loss of our house, due to financial difficulties, I discovered a sort of lump on my right breast. I immediately rushed to my family doctor who plainly told me to get an appointment with a surgeon. It was obvious to me that this lump was cancerous. I scheduled an appointment with a surgeon at my neighborhood hospital and after x-rays and tests, my surgeon concluded that I had a hormone-related tumor. After surgery, he suggested I should undergo hormonal therapy.

With the help of my daughter, Alexia, who was employed by a big pharmaceutical company in France, I got a second opinion at the UCSF breast cancer center in San Francisco, which is well known for its latest research.

There, the head of the breast cancer department, Dr. Rugo, ordered some more x-rays and tests and it was discovered that I had two different tumors in the same breast that were very aggressive Stage 3. She recommended chemotherapy before surgery to eradicate the tumors and if the chemotherapy worked, I would then have a lumpectomy followed by radiotherapy. I started six months of chemotherapy in November 2011, a time much delayed due to the amount of research to determine the best treatment. Treatment occurred once a week and lasted for five hours. For me, it was not painful nor difficult to bear but the only thing that I disliked was a feeling of wasted time and the pungent smell of drugs in the infusion center.

After five months of chemotherapy and two months of radiotherapy, my tumors decreased enough to receive surgery. I was even lucky enough to avoid a mastectomy and after a bit of reconstructive surgery, found myself feeling more youthful and attractive. After another five years of hormone therapy, a move back to my roots in France, and the birth of my grandson, Alexia's baby, I have been in complete remission.

I consider myself very lucky to have gone through chemotherapy without being extremely tired or sick. I led a calmer life while going through cancer than I used to beforehand, resting during the day and walking every afternoon. I ate well and complimented my diet with a variety of supplements.

In spite of that, several unexpected problems occurred during treatment, the first being my port that had to be removed, as it had caused some blood clots in my jugular vein. The port could have really put my life in danger if my body didn't react instinctively by waking me during the middle of the night with such pain that I asked to go to the hospital. The blood clots were discovered with a full scan and I went home after a shot of anticoagulant and a prescription for two months of treatment. After this episode, the nurses had to do the IVs directly through the vein in my arm instead of through a port. This was a very delicate process as the medicine was so corrosive that it could damage the arm forever if the liquid spread outside the vein. I also had to have blood transfusions several times because my blood count had become abnormal.

A funny story to share is an incident which happened with my wig which I wore after the loss of my hair. I could never perfect putting my wig on my head the correct way. So, one day, the postman came to the door and when I opened the door, a gust of wind sent the wig flying off my head onto the floor. The postman was so astonished to witness this he even apologized.

After the chemotherapy sessions, which succeeded in completely removing the tumors, I underwent a lumpectomy. After the surgery healed, I was scheduled for radiotherapy, every week for two-month sessions. However, the radiotherapy had to be delayed as my mother passed away in France and I had to fly to attend her funeral.

To conclude, I really don't think breast cancer was a disease that could have possibly ended my life. It was purely an unpleasant experience I had to go through. I never experienced the side effects that most patients endure, and I generally even refused the medicines that were offered, as I didn't need them. Besides resting and exercising every day, I took advantage of the numerous conferences and advice offered at the hospital and elsewhere. Now, after six years have passed, I feel fine and cancer seems far away, a distant memory. I do go for checkups every year and get mammograms, blood tests and bone density tests. I stopped taking Letrozole and I am hoping to reach my 10-year cancer remission marker which I'm sure I can achieve.

Christine's story written by her daughter, Alexia:
My mother, Christine, had just turned 71 years old and was struggling with a lot of worries and trauma prior to her diagnosis. She had lost her mother to a choking incident and she had also lost her younger sister to an embolism which caused her to have a fatal stroke in her bathtub. I was 35 years old at the time living in France and experiencing fertility problems and my mother and her husband were facing financial difficulties.

One day my mother noticed she was feeling tension in her right breast. "With all of this stress I feel like I'm going to get cancer again," she said to me. When she was 35 years old and pregnant with me, she had almost died from Melanoma skin cancer in 1997.

The family pushed my mother to go in for a checkup and that's when she found out she had a double tumor in her right breast. She was diagnosed with stage 3 breast cancer. This new diagnosis brought back upsetting memories from her past and everyone was in shock, especially when she announced she wanted to try to treat her cancer without chemotherapy or Western medicine.

During this time I was working at a pharmaceutical company in France. My colleagues called UCSF in San Francisco where they were partnering on a clinical trial that covered my mother's type of cancer and age range. UCSF was able to get my mother on the clinical trial list in San Francisco.

At first, my mother was reluctant to go ahead with the trial, but with a little push from our friends and family, and after researching the odds of surviving cancer by only changing her diet, doing enemas and natural treatments, she decided to take part in the trial. I looked into taking a sabbatical from work to travel from San Francisco to support my mother during her journey to what she hoped would be a full recovery.

I accompanied my mother to the day-long chemotherapy sessions. This is when we befriended Hillary who was going through a similar treatment plan. My mother and Hillary were able to share experiences, their ups and downs, and bonded by sharing stories about their past and travels. Having an emotional support system is probably one of the most essential factors for being able to cope with the treatments and heal from cancer. The relationship that my mother and Hillary formed going through this process together certainly gave them that extra strength and was invaluable in staying positive and surviving cancer.

My mother luckily dealt with the side effects of chemotherapy rather well. She didn't experience nausea and pain, however, she was alarmed and depressed when her hair came out in bundles on the pillow. I took her to get her head shaved and called the resourceful Breast Cancer Society who provided free wigs and also therapy sessions with a social worker.

My mother did have other issues to face during her treatment that were life-threatening. She got an infection around her port and had to get several blood transfusions which made her very weak.

It was a scary time for the whole family. My mother knew that by changing her diet to exclude meat, coffee, and sugar and increase regular exercise, specifically walking, she would be able to better cope with a foggy brain, fatigue and mood swings from the chemo and increase her chances of survival.

I learned by being a caregiver to my mother that having a cancer diagnosis can feel overwhelming and stressful not only for the person who has to endure the illness but also for their loved ones. I also learned that having a strong emotional support system and believing in a positive outcome helps get through the obstacles and pain and ultimately gives one strength to be able to lead a more fruitful life.

Through being a caregiver to my mother I realized that I wanted to use my optimism and positive outlook on life to inspire and nurture the idea that with the right mindset, attitude and resources everything is possible. After my mother recovered, I became a life coach and to this day strive to raise my clients' awareness about their strengths, aspirations and potential as well as behaviors and underlying motives for change. Exploring and working through fears, assumptions and limiting beliefs about oneself and others allows you to identify new ways that you can use your strength in the workplace and in relationships. As I found it rewarding to support my mother through her cancer experience, I do my best to support others now in their journey making personal visions a reality.

Daphne

Daphne and I met in high school at a small girls' boarding school outside Boston in the Berkshires. Our friendship is a lifelong friendship which began in 1983. We were on the same tennis team and were fairly close in school but we became closer friends when we both moved to San Francisco and discovered we were living in the same back yard. We also both gave birth to two children in the same order around the same time and bonded in the experience of becoming new mothers.

In 2008 my daughter and I were invited to her daughter Eleanor's four-year-old magical Cinderella princess themed birthday party with a real-live singing and performing Cinderella which the adults enjoyed as much as the children. When my in-laws visited San Francisco from England, Daphne and her husband Mike were always gracious, inviting our family over for dinner. Both Rudi Sr. and Mike were avid sailors and bonded, recounting sailing stories as well as sailing together on the San Francisco Bay.

Around the same time I was coming out of treatment, Daphne's mother, Stefanie, was diagnosed with lung cancer in 2012. After going through treatment myself, I understood what this was like and stepped in to deliver soup, a meal and heartfelt support. Daphne was also one of the caregivers in her family who helped her mother through treatment and supported her move out to California, through independent living in San Francisco to assisted care. Daphne was grateful to have two additional years with her mother from what the doctors initially expected. Stefanie Jackson passed away August 2014 with her daughter Daphne by her side.

Four years went by after her mother's passing and unexpectedly, Daphne was diagnosed with Non-Hodgkin's Lymphoma in December 2017 at the age of 49. The reflections she shares here on guilt, competitiveness and the gift of cancer are insightful, authentic, real, witty, and heartfelt.

Daphne writes:
The particular cancer diagnosis of non-Hodgkins Lymphoma, can be

confusing. It has the two big, ugly "c's"- cancer and chemotherapy. But, as someone said to me once, "It's like the flu: it used to kill us and now it doesn't." Meaning there is a tried and true treatment for it which I'm utterly grateful. The word "curable" is a rare term to use with cancer patients and due to its curability, I felt guilty.

The guilt came in wondering if I deserved the same empathy, help, and amazing kindness of family, friends and acquaintances that cancer patients need to receive. The same attention as patients with riskier, more tenuous diagnoses. I felt guilty receiving all the concern, time and attention, because I knew I was going to get through my cancer, according to the statistics. There are friends who have chronic diseases that are far less visible, but at times can be just as debilitating, diseases that require a lifetime of understanding, help and compassion from friends and family, and they don't always receive the support they need.

But NHL is not the flu, and it doesn't feel like the flu. It's not like anything I'd ever felt before. It's not pain; you feel like the sludge at the bottom of a boat's bilge. It maybe is "curable," but it's still cancer and it's still chemotherapy. The journey is real: the myriad of endless doctor's appointments, registrations, check-ups, needles, nausea, hair loss, low white blood cell counts, lack of energy, curtailed schedule, anxiety, deterioration of bodily functions, physical and emotional roller coaster. It will change you, you may be cured, but you will always be looking over your shoulder because it's cancer. This is not the flu.

Over time, I came to see that guilt is unhealthy and cheats you of the full healing power of community and kindness. Toward the end of my treatment, I finally learned to express gratitude without guilt: to just soak in the kindness as intended. I also trusted that I could and would be able to pay-it-forward.

Competitiveness

A common refrain I heard when I told people I was going through cancer treatment was, "Oh, my friend has the exact same thing and did so well!" My immediate reaction was, "Am I doing well?" While intending to be supportive, I came to realize no one has the exact same thing or certainly not the exact same experience because everyone's body is different, different ages, stages, different immune systems, different pre-existing conditions, different emotional hurdles...the list goes on.

I spent an inordinately ridiculous amount of time and energy trying to figure out if I was "doing this well." Am I down "the fairway" in terms of my reaction to chemo or am I having outlier reactions, more tired than others, more inflammation pain than others? It's not an issue of being a hypochondriac, it comes from the need to compare if I'm "good at this." Complaining too much or being strong? It doesn't matter how you are responding relatively; you are the make and model that you are and worrying about where you are on "the spectrum" is very unproductive.

I realized sometime after the first or second treatment that I didn't need to "sail through" this with accolades. I didn't need to be someone's extraordinary or impressive story about how well I coped with the treatment. I didn't need to be notable, extra brave or heroic. There was no one's admiration I had to win or pat on the head for "doing it well." I just needed to get better, and try to juggle a few balls along the way. Keep just a few things moving forward that seemed to be most needed. Try to normalize family life.

It's how and when you heal that is all that matters. If you don't feel like crap, then you should worry. Chemo is doing its job when it kills the fastest growing cells, all of them everywhere in your body, hopefully getting all the bad ones first. Hair, nails, lungs, heart, liver, intestines, nerve endings, whatever. Chemo works when these hurt.

Where does the need to be "doing this well" come from? I don't want to take up too much space with my illness? Be too much of an imposition? What insecurity has this exposed? What can I learn from this about myself? It's exposing an almost debilitating desire to "be good" and now I'm trying to be good at being sick (Please Laugh!). I know I'm not unique in this. I believe mothers today, in particular, feel the pressure to be doing everything well at the exact same time. Let it go. Let lots of things go. All your internal energy should be focused on feeling as good as you can about yourself.

The Gift
Gifts can emerge from times of crisis; things that give the struggle a sense of purpose or meaning. People told me to be open, but I didn't see it . . . until I finally did.

The Gift was my daughter and I didn't see this one coming at all. A very large part of my relationship with Eleanor over the years has been struggling with her intense range of emotions, coping with her frustrations, usually released towards me. It's been a journey for our family to live with and unpack this part of her personality. How to manage it, respond to it, coach her out of it, not react to it, give her tools to understand her emotions and constantly find new ways to manage them as she grew. We always showed her unconditional love and support and stayed open and encouraging when progress was being made. At age 12 and 13, she meaningfully started to turn a corner.

Something happened when I got sick. Our roles switched. I had to let go, and she had to step forward. She saw how imperfect and vulnerable I was; how I looked without hair, that I had to slow way down and sleep a lot. The Saturday I was throwing up. The Friday I had a fever of 103.5. She realized she could help me by taking care of herself; that she could make me feel better, and that I needed her help.

Eleanor would often ask me how I'm doing with a very sweet, sincerely concerned voice that would catch me off-guard and melt my heart always after a treatment day. She tracked my treatments, knew which number it was and found me as soon as she got home. She realized she could really help me. It helped her get out of her head, gave her a role, gave her some control. Eleanor would make her own breakfast, her school lunch and often the same for her brother. She would make me tea and breakfasts in bed. She would loosely track what I ate and tell me to eat more. She wrote me lovely notes and brought flowers.

Eleanor developed a caregiver's patience, kindness and restraint. She also seemed to start trusting me more. My being sick and vulnerable made me more accessible and approachable for her; humanized me more. Eleanor is a deeply empathetic person, one of her many amazing characteristics, and this experience let her see me through that lens. It was Eleanor who said "Mom, you wear hats and scarves all the time, but you know you can "rock the bald look." That felt liberating and empowering. We both felt a profound change then and now. Me letting go, Eleanor stepping forward and forever changing the tenor of our relationship.

Sonja

I met Sonja Faulkner, Ph.D. through Hope. In 1949, when my mother was 16 years old and Hope's father, Brooks, was 18 years old Brooks helped my mother's family with roof work at their Pound Ridge New York farm. Fast forward to July 2007, the year after my father passed away my mother was feeling lonely and decided to look up Brooks' phone number through the directory. She found him in Holden, Maine. Brooks was surprised and pleased to hear from my mother and they soon after started a long-distance relationship. Brooks spoke to my mother every single day for 19 months on the phone and even visited her in Florida four times. Tragically, in February 2009 Brooks went into the hospital in Bangor, Maine for a prostate operation but he never recovered. Brooks passed after his surgery on February 24, 2009 at the age of 77.

His daughter, Hope, was the gift to our family. Hope is warm and gracious and stayed close to our family. Hope's close friend, Sonja sent me the book she wrote when I was going through treatment, *The Best Friend's Guide to Breast Cancer*. The interconnectivity in life is a beautiful thing to experience.

Sonja wrote:
Many people will probably mention yoga, meditation, eating well, exercise, aromatherapy, or any number of other alternative therapies that help during a cancer battle. All of these modalities deserve our attention and discussion, but I'd like to give a shout out to something else that I believe is profoundly and universally therapeutic.

I've spent the past eight years or so telling anyone who would listen that the healing power of social support is extraordinary: "As the friend, loved one, co-worker, or acquaintance of someone facing cancer, know that you have the power to make a significant difference in their life!" I believe this with every cell in my body. But what I've learned is that it goes both ways—it's wonderful to offer support; it's also healing to accept it. If you've been diagnosed with cancer, my hope is that you'll let people in. Even if you're fiercely independent and not the type who likes to ask anything of others (my hand is raised right there with you!), try to let your guard down a bit at this time. People want to help. Let them. If a support group isn't your thing, that's okay. It doesn't need to be a formal gathering. The point is to open your mind and heart and accept the love, support, and kindness that people extend to you. The healing power of these meaningful acts is tremendous.

I have one more slice of insight I'd like to share. There's a whole rainbow of reactions to a cancer diagnosis, which may include fear, sadness, confusion, and just generally being pissed off at the world. Any feeling is yours, and make no mistake, you're entitled to it. With that said, though, I'd encourage those facing cancer to keep a gratitude journal. The past is gone and the future is uncertain, even for those who don't have cancer. All we have is now. So try to focus your mind on the present and jot down the things that make you smile or bring a tear of thankfulness to your eyes—perhaps how nice that cold ice cream feels on your throat that's raw and blistered from chemotherapy or radiation...or the softness of a cozy blanket that envelops you in warmth and comfort...or that you were able to keep some food down at lunch today...or a friend who gave you a hearty belly laugh, even though you felt like hell...or a sweet, gentle kiss from a loved one, with a knowing look of understanding that transcends the situation...or the wonderful surprise of a pal from your distant past who reached out to let you know that she was thinking about you. The list is endless, limited only by our inability to appreciate even the littlest moments of beauty.

No one would dispute that cancer is a wretched disease. But if you open your heart to the kindness and support all around you, it can make your journey unexpectedly exquisite. I wish all of my cancer sisters and brothers light, love, and healing.

No one is free from their inevitable death

Peter Fenwick's work on the dying process, specifically his TedX talk and book, *The Art of Dying,* helped me understand the natural process around death. My friend and former colleague, Nigel, was warm and funny and we used to joke and laugh together in the office. He had liver cancer and we were keeping in touch by email. He approached his death with bravery and a sense of peace. I want to close with Nigel's endearing email to me right before he passed.

May 25, 2015

My Dear Fellow Fighter,

Forgive me but I am beginning to lose this particular battle. I have had two horrible operations on my liver this calendar year and have recently spent a couple of weeks in the hospital. I was sent home a couple of days ago because there was no more they could do for me. To wake in my own bed, with my family close by is a marvelous experience. I am not too sure how long the next phase lasts. We have both laughed a great deal over the years, and that is how I want you to remember me.

Much love, xx

Nigel Jones

"Row, row, row your boat
Gently down the stream
Merrily, merrily, merrily, merrily
Life is but a dream."

PART VII

ACKNOWLEDGMENTS

Each friend represents a world in us,
a world possibly not born until they arrive,
and it is only by this meeting that a new world is born.

– Anais Nin

Thank you to all my caring friends and my family near and far for all of your support through my cancer diagnosis and treatment. I owe a lot to so many people but I would like to thank the following for their love, support and encouragement in writing my book:

The Wellness Seed:
Jumbe Allen
Dr. Sarah Kalomiros
Bob Bearden
Leslie Smith
Rudolf John Polednik
Cornelia Elwood
Amy Maier
Leah San Souci
Jennifer Valentyn

Alexia, Anna, Anne, Betsy G, Betsy J., Betsy S., Brian, Caren, Carman, Cathy, Cecilia, Christine, Daphne, Deirdre, Eimile, Eliza, Elizabeth P., Elie, Ellen, Elona, Eva (Aunt), Faith, Fitz, Forrest, Gabrielle, Gail R., Gail (Mom), Greta, Heidi, Hope, Jane, Jasper, Jeannie, Jen P., Jen W., Joyce, Judy, Julia, Julie, Justine, Karen, Karin, Kirsten, Laura, Laurie P., Laurie S., Leslie L., Lindsey, Lisa L, Lisa O., Liz P., Lucy B., Lucy S., Mai Mai, Marci, Margarita, Marie Jo, Mary, May, Melissa, Merideth, Miranda, Michael B., Michael H., Monica, Monique, Naomi, Nicole, Nina, Peter, Randa, Rhys, Sarah, Sasha, Seson, Sonja, Stephanie L, Stephanie S., Susan, Susie, Suz, Tam, Terry, Tess G., Tomas, Vini, Zarina

I am grateful to my editor for believing in me and for her support and guidance in this project:
Sally Wolfe

Publisher:
Gary Revel

Designer:
Jennifer Valentyn

In Fond Memory:
Allen Hartley Seed
Rudolf Milan Polednik
Brooks Mills
Renee Heidtman
Nigel Jones
Dorothy Divack
Ray Nowakowski
Peyton McKeehan
Silvina Nieves Meshel
Mia Oliver
Sydney Stone
Louise Hay
Wayne Dyer
Beloved Animals - Holly, Lola, Harvey & Lulu

PART VIII
ABOUT THE AUTHOR

Hillary Polednik lives in San Francisco with her husband, Rudi. She is a devoted Mom to two teenagers and two guinea pigs. Hillary went through breast cancer in June 2011 at the age of 45. She was inspired to write about her cancer journey to help others in their healing process in this creative, self-help memoir.

Hillary grew up outside of Boston and attended Wheaton College in Norton, Massachusetts, graduating in 1989 where she majored in studio art and won the Mariam F. Carpenter Art Award.

Hillary is also an Account Executive in telecommunications and is passionate about bridging the gap between technology and the holistic health and wellness mind-body-spirit world.

You can visit her website:

www.TheWellnessSeed.com

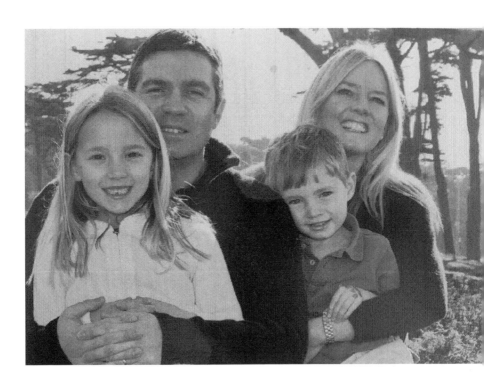

Hillary and Family

PART IX

THE WELLNESS SEED RESOURCE CHECK LIST

Health is a state of complete harmony of the body, mind and spirit. When one is free from physical disabilities and mental distraction, the gates of the soul open.

B.K.S. Lyengar

Health and wellness information is abundant everywhere you turn, especially on the internet. This sample list of resources has been collected and reviewed to help you make the best choices for yourself or a loved one. One way to make the best use of the following resources is to review the list and check boxes you are attracted to and then follow up with your own inquiry or research.

Sources, books, and websites are provided as information only. I have found these resources helpful and recommend them to you as part of your healing journey. Often it's not just one person or one resource that helps you on your healing journey, it's the input and knowledge of the collective consciousness - whether doctors, nutritionists, massage therapists, acupuncturists, spiritual counselors, authors, holistic health and wellness practitioners, thought leaders, colleagues, family and friends, and also importantly the intuition and guidance of your own self. The goal from the collective is to empower yourself by gaining knowledge and to create a strong supportive community on your road to recovery.

ALTERNATIVE CANCER TREATMENT - HOSPITALS AND CLINICS

☐ Burzynski Clinic | Houston TX | www.burzynskiclinic.com

☐ CMN Hospital | San Luis Rio Colorado Mexico | www.cmnact.com

☐ Sanoviv Medical Institute | Baja Mexico | www.sanoviv.com

DOCTORS – WELLNESS

☐ Dr. Josh Axe | www.draxe.com

☐ Dr. Neal D. Barnard | www.pcrm.org

☐ Dr. David Brownstein | www.drbrownstein.com

☐ Dr. T. Colin Campbell | www.beatcancer.org

☐ Dr. William Courtney | www.cannabisinternational.org

☐ Dr. Gabriel Cousens | www.treeoflifecenterus.com

☐ Dr. Larry Dossey | www.dosseydossey.com

☐ Dr. Isaac Eliaz | www.dreliaz.com

☐ Dr. Caldwell Esselstyn | www.dresselstyn.com

☐ Dr. Joel Fuhrman | www.drfuhrman.com

☐ Dr. Michael Greger | www.drgreger.org

☐ Dr. Christine Horner| www.drchristinehorner.com

☐ Dr. Mark Hyman | www.drhyman.com

☐ Dr. Joel S. Kahn | www.drjoelkahn.com

☐ Dr. David Katz | www.davidkatzmd.com

☐ Dr. Michael Klaper | www.doctorklaper.com

☐ Dr. Frank Lipman | www.drfranklipman.com

☐ Dr. Robert Lustig | www.robertlustig.com

- ☐ Dr. John A. McDougall | www.mcdougall.com
- ☐ Dr. Joseph Mercola | www.mercola.com
- ☐ Dr. Christine Northrup | www.drnorthrup.com
- ☐ Dr. Dean Ornish | www.deanornish.com
- ☐ Dr. David Perlmutter | www.drperlmutter.com
- ☐ Dr. Alona Pulde | www.forksoverknives.com
- ☐ Dr. Lissa Rankin | www.lissarankin.com
- ☐ Dr. Bernie Siegel | www.berniesiegelmd.com
- ☐ Dr. Terry Wahls | www.terrywahls.com
- ☐ Dr. Andrew Weil | www.drweil.com
- ☐ Dr. Bruce West | www.healthalert.com

FIND A FUNCTIONAL, INTEGRATIVE OR NATUROPATHIC DOCTOR

- ☐ The Institute for Functional Medicine | www.ifm.org
- ☐ Find an integrative physician "near you" | www.acam.org
- ☐ Online naturopathic physicians | www.naturopathichealth.net

MEDICAL CARE WEBSITE

- ☐ Find best medical care website | www.idealmedicalcare.org

SAFE BEAUTY PRODUCTS

ELIMINATE ENVIRONMENTAL TOXINS

☐ Center for Environmental Health | www.ceh.org

☐ Environmental Working Group Skin Deep | www.ewg.org

Check your ingredients for your body and home: beauty product - body cream, soap, shampoo, conditioner, deodorant, hand soap, sunscreen, also home products: cleaning supplies, dish soap, laundry detergent - throw out cosmetics with chemicals and also subscribe to Environmental Working Group for the latest health information.

☐ Sustainable living tips | www.sustainablebabysteps.com

ESSENTIAL OILS TO HELP WITH CANCER

☐ Frankincense

☐ Lavender

☐ Palo Santo

☐ Valerian

☐ Ylang Ylang

ESSENTIAL OIL BRANDS

☐ Aura Cacia | www.auracacia.com

☐ DoTERRA | www.doterra.com

☐ Edens Garden | www.edensgarden.com

☐ Plant Therapy Essential oils | www.planttherapy.com

☐ Rocky Mountain oils | www.rockymountainoils.com

☐ Young Living | www.youngliving.com

PERSONAL CARE

☐ Think Dirty app | Scan barcodes in the grocery store with your phone to get a reading on what beauty products are clean. www.thinkdirtyapp.com

SAFE COSMETICS

☐ 100% Pure | www.100percentpure.com

☐ Aubrey Organics | www.aubreyorganics.com

☐ Bare Minerals by Bare Escentuals | www.bareescentuals.com

☐ Beauty Counter | www.beautycounter.com

☐ Burts Bees | www.burtsbees.com

☐ Colorescience | www.colorescience.com

☐ DermOrganic | www.dermorganic.com

☐ Dr. Bronner's | www.drbronner.com

☐ Eco Bella | www.eccobella.com

☐ Eminence | www.eminenceorganics.com

☐ EO Products | www.eoproducts.com

☐ Evan Healy | www.evanhealy.com

☐ Goop | www.goop.com

☐ Jane Iredale | www.janeiredale.com

☐ John Masters Organics | www.johnmasters.com

☐ Juice Beauty | www.juicebeauty.com

☐ Jurilique | www.jurilique.com

☐ Kiss My Face | www.kissmyface.com

☐ La Bella Donna Mineral Make-up | www.labelladonna.com

☐ Luzern Laboratories | www.luzernlabs.com

☐ Mineral Fusion | www.mineralfusion.com

☐ Neil's Yard Remedies | www.nealsyardremedies.com

☐ Pangea Organics | www.pangeaorganics.com

☐ Real Purity | www.realpurity.com

☐ RMS Beauty | www.rmsbeauty.com

CANCER INFORMATION

☐ Breast Cancer blog | www.keep-a-breast.org

☐ Cancer Tutor website | www.cancertutor.com

☐ Center for New Medicine | www.cfnmedcine.com

☐ Chris Wark | Chris Beat Cancer |www.chrisbeatcancer.com

☐ Dr. Kelly Turner | www.drkellyturner.com

☐ Dr. Servan-Schreiber's Story | www.anticancerbook.com

☐ Nancy's List | Austin TX | Cancer stories and countrywide resources list | nancyslist.org

☐ Radical Remission Project | www.radicalremission.com

☐ Ty Bolinger | The Truth About Cancer www.thetruthaboutcancer.com

COUNSELING

FIND A LIFE COACH, HOLISTIC HEALTH AND WELLNESS COACH

☐ BetterUp | www.betterup.com

☐ Google search | Life Coach | Wellness Health Coach "near me"

☐ Yelp | Life Coach | Wellness Health Coach "in name of your city"

FIND A LICENSED MENTAL | EMOTIONAL THERAPIST

☐ 7CupsofTea | www.7cups.com

☐ Betterhelp | www.betterhelp.com

☐ Breakthrough | www.breakthrough.com

☐ MyTherapist| www.mytherapist.com

☐ TalkSpace | www.talkspace.com

☐ Google search | Licensed Therapist "near me"

☐ Yelp | Licensed Therapist "in name of your city"

ONLINE CANCER SUPPORT GROUP MATCHES

☐ Cancer Hope Network | www.cancerhopenetwork.org

☐ Google search | Online cancer support group "in name of your city"

MEET UP WITH A COMMUNITY OF LIKE-MINDED OTHERS

☐ Join a community at Meetup | www.meetup.com

FAMILY SUPPORT CARE CALENDARS

☐ CaringBridge | Personal health journal that keep friends and family up to date with health updates | www.caringbridge.com

☐ MyLifeLine | Social and emotional support services for cancer patients | www.mylifeline.org

MOVEMENT

EXERCISE IDEAS

☐ Aerobic class

☐ Badminton

☐ Barre Method

☐ Basketball

☐ Biking

☐ Bocce Ball

☐ Boot camp

☐ Bowling

☐ Chi Gong

☐ Croquet

☐ Cross country skiing

☐ Dancing

☐ Downhill skiing

☐ Elliptical

☐ Field Hockey

☐ Football

- ☐ Frisbee
- ☐ Golfing
- ☐ Grounding-walk barefoot
- ☐ Gym
- ☐ Hiking
- ☐ Home stretching
- ☐ Ice skating
- ☐ Jump roping
- ☐ Karate
- ☐ Kayak
- ☐ Kick boxing
- ☐ Lift weights
- ☐ Martial Arts
- ☐ Paddle tennis
- ☐ Paddleboard
- ☐ Personal trainer
- ☐ Pilates
- ☐ Rebounder trampoline
- ☐ Rock Climbing
- ☐ Rowing
- ☐ Running
- ☐ Scuba Diving
- ☐ Snorkel

- ☐ Snowshoeing

- ☐ Soccer

- ☐ Spinning class

- ☐ Stationary bike

- ☐ Surfing

- ☐ Swimming

- ☐ Tai Chi

- ☐ Tennis

- ☐ Treadmill

- ☐ Vibration plate

- ☐ Volleyball

- ☐ Walking

- ☐ Water polo

- ☐ Windsurfing

- ☐ Yoga

YOGA STUDIOS

- ☐ Moxie | www.moxie.yoga

- ☐ Ritual Hot Yoga | www.ritualhotyoga.com

- ☐ The Mindful Body | www.themindfulbody.com

- ☐ Yoga Flow San Francisco | www.yogaflowsf.com

- ☐ Google search | Yoga studios "near me"

- ☐ Yelp | Yoga studios "in name of your city"

MASSAGE

☐ International Orange | www.intenationalorange.com

☐ Kabuki Spa & Springs | www.kabukisprings.com

☐ Nob Hill Spa | www.nobhillspa.com

☐ Pearl Spa & Sauna | www.pearlspasf.com

☐ Sen Spa | www.senspa.com

☐ Spa Radiance | www.sparadiance.com

☐ Google search | Massage "near me"

☐ Yelp | Massage "in name of your city"

REIKI ENERGY HEALING

☐ Robert Bearden | Healing Happens

☐ Marci Baron | www.marcibaronclears.com

☐ Google search | Reiki "near me"

☐ Yelp | Reiki "in name of your city"

INFRARED SAUNA SPAS

☐ Sen Spa | www.senspa.com

☐ Reboot Float & Cryotherapy Spa | www.rebootfloatspa.com

☐ Google search | Infrared sauna "near me"

☐ Yelp | Infrared sauna "in name of your city"

INFRARED SAUNA – TO BUY

☐ Sauna Works | Clearlight Infrared Sauna | www.infraredsauna.com

☐ Sauna Cloud Infrared Saunas | www.saunacloud.com

☐ Google search | Infrared Sauna to "buy near me"

MIND AND MEDITATION

☐ Barry Michels | Tools to access creative power of unconscious
www.thetoolsbook.com

☐ Charlie Knowles | The Veda Center for Meditation
www.thevedacenter.com

☐ Dharma Seed Buddhist Vipassana | www.dharmasseed.org

☐ Dr. Joe Dispenza Rewiring Your Brain | www.drjoedispenza.com

☐ Dr. Marty Rossman | Anxiety Help | www.thehealingmind.org

☐ Finerminds | Personal growth | www.finerminds.com

☐ "I Am" positive emotions | www.paulsantisimeditations.com

☐ Institute of Noetic Sciences (IONS) | www.noetic.org

☐ Mind Body Spirit courses | www.mindvalleyacademy.com

☐ Mind Valley | www.mindvalley.com

☐ Pema Chödrön Foundation | www.pemachodronfoundation.org

☐ Rick Hanson, Ph.D. | www.rickhanson.net

☐ Rob William's Psych-K Centre International | www.psych-k.com

☐ Spirit Rock Meditation Center | www.spiritrock.org

☐ The Amen Clinics | Brain health | www.amenclinics.com

MEDITATION CLASS

☐ Google search | Meditation class "near me"

☐ Yelp | Meditation class "in name of your city"

MEDITATION APPS

☐ Aura | www.aurahealth.io

☐ Calm | www.calm.com

☐ Headspace | www.headspace.com

☐ Insight Timer | www.insighttimer.com

☐ Smiling Mind | www.smilingmind.com.au

☐ Stop, Breathe & Think | www.stopbreathethink.com

☐ Ten Percent Happier | www.tenpercent.com

BREATHING APP

☐ The Breathing App

☐ Stop, Breathe & Think

☐ Breathing Zone

☐ Prana Breath: Calm & Meditate

☐ Breathe Easy App

☐ Universal Breathing: Pranayama

HEALTH APPS

☐ 8Fit | Workouts and meal planner

☐ Fooducate | Improve health with a real food diet

☐ MyFitnessPal | Tracking and motivation

☐ SleepCycle | Intelligent alarm clock analyzes sleep

☐ Stand Up! | Flexible work break timer

WELLNESS TOOLS TO TRANSFORM YOUR LIFE

☐ eMindful | Online mindfulness courses | www.emindful.com

EFT – EMOTIONAL FREEDOM TECHNIQUE

☐ The Tapping Solution | www.thetappingsolution.com

ACUPUNCTURE

☐ Chinese Medicine Works | www.chinesemedicineworks.com

☐ Google search | Acupuncture "near me"

☐ Yelp | Acupuncture "in name of your city"

HOLISTIC HEALTH

☐ Ayurveda information | www.joyfulbelly.com

☐ Free cancer guide on holistic health | www.trulyheal.com

☐ Mike Adams "Health Ranger" | www.healthranger.com

☐ Google search | Holistic health coach "near me"

FIND A HOLISTIC DENTIST

☐ Holistic Dental Association | www.holisticdental.org

☐ Dental Wellness Institute | www.dentalwellness4u.com

☐ Google search | Holistic dentist "near me"

☐ Yelp | Holistic dentist "in name of your city"

DIRECTORY OF BIOLOGICAL DENTISTS

☐ Directory of Biological Dentists | www.iabdm.org

☐ Mercury free Biological Dentist | www.talkinternational.com

INTERNATIONAL ACADEMY OF ORAL MEDICINE | TOXICOLOGY

☐ International Academy of Oral Medicine & Toxicology
www.iaomt.org

LAB SERVICES & HEALTH EVALUATIONS

☐ 23andme | Saliva test for gene testing | www.23andme.com

☐ Livewello | Health gene report | www.livewello.com

☐ Self Decode | Personalized health report | www.selfdecode.com

☐ ZRT Laboratories | Saliva test for hormone evaluation periodically
www.zrtlab.com

MEDICAL MARIJUANA

☐ Rick Simpson | Cannabis oil | www.phoenixtears.ca

☐ Medical Marijuana | Delivery to your door | www.eaze.com

☐ Jetty Extracts | Cannabis | www.jettyextracts.com

☐ Google search | Medical marijuana "near me"

☐ Yelp | Medical marijuana "in name of your city"

CBD OIL AND MEDICAL MARIJUANA

☐ The Apothecarium | www.apothecarium.com

☐ Cole Street Smoke Shop | www.sanfranciscosmokeshop.com

☐ The Green Cross | www.thegreencross.org

☐ Harvest | www.harvestshop.com

☐ NuggMD | www.getnugg.com

☐ Urban Pharm | www.up415.com

☐ Bloom Room | www.bloomroom.com

☐ Barbary Coast | www.barbarycoastsf.org

☐ Google search | CBD oil "near me"

☐ Yelp | CBD oil "in name of your city"

NUTRITION

NUTRITION - GENERAL

☐ Nutrition information Dr. Price | www.westonaprice.org

☐ The Gluten Summit | www.theglutensummit.com

☐ Ocean Robbins | www.oceanrobbins.com

☐ Mark Sisson | Mark's Daily Apple | www.marksdailyapple.com

☐ Dr. McDougall's Medical Center | www.drmcdougall.com

☐ NutritionFacts | www.nutritionfacts.org

☐ Plant-based nutrition healthcare conference | www.pbnhc.com

☐ Center for Nutrition Studies | www.nutritionstudies.org

☐ Life Extension Nutrient test | www.lef.org

☐ Healthy Plant-based eating | www.21dayveganblueprint.com

☐ Institute for Responsible Nutrition | www.responsiblefoods.org

☐ GreenMedInfo | www.greenmedinfo.com

☐ The Plant Based Dietitian | www.plantbaseddietitian.com

☐ Thrivemarket | www.thrivemarket.com

☐ Gerson Diet | www.gerson.org

☐ Alkaline diet | www.thealkalinediet.com

☐ Earth Clinic | www.earthclinic.com

☐ Trudy Scott, CN | www.antianxietyfoodsolution.com

NUTRITIONISTS

☐ Core Care Center | www.corecarecenter.com

☐ Dr. Thomas Cowen | www.fourfoldhealing.com

☐ Institute for Health and Healing | www.sutterhealth.org

☐ Trudy Scott CN | www.antianxietyfoodsolution.com

☐ Google search | Nutritionists | Nutritionist "near me"

☐ Yelp | Nutritionists | Nutritionist "in name of your city"

COOKBOOKS

☐ Cancer Fighting Kitchen by Rebecca Katz

☐ Dr. Mercola's Total Health Cookbook by Dr. Joseph Mercola

☐ Getting into Food by Allison Imel-Hamza

☐ Gluten-Free Girl by Shana James Ahren

☐ Healthy Gluten-Free Cooking by Darina Allen & Rosemary Kearney

☐ Jamie's Food Revolution by Jamie Oliver

☐ Local Flavors, cooking and eating from America's farmers
by Deborah Madison

☐ Nourishing Traditions by Sally Fallon

☐ Recipes For Longer Life by Ann Wigmore

☐ Roots by Diane Morgan

☐ Straight from the Earth cookbook by Myra Goodman

☐ Super Natural Every Day by Heidi Swanson

☐ The Garden of Eating – A Produce Dominated Diet
by Rachel Albert-Matesz

☐ The Food of Life by Versatile Vegetable

☐ The Primal Blueprint Cookbook by Mark Sisson

☐ The Victory Garden Cookbook by Marian Morash

☐ The Whole Life Nutrition by Alissa Segersten & Tom Malterre

☐ Truly Cultured by Nancy Lee Bentley

☐ Wild Fermentation by Sandor Elliz Katz

HEALTHY GROCERY STORES

☐ Mollie Stone's Market | www.molliestones.com

☐ Rainbow Grocery | www.rainbow.coop

☐ Real Food Company | www.realfoodco.com

☐ Trader Joe's | www.traderjoes.com

☐ Whole Foods Market | www.wholefoodsmarket.com

ONLINE ORGANIC GROCERIES AND RECIPES

☐ Nutiva | www.nutiva.com

☐ Planet Organics | www.planetorganics.com

PERSONAL CHEF SERVICES

☐ Taylored Taste | Lucy Bowen Tayor | lucybowen@yahoo.com

☐ Google search | Personal chef "near me"

☐ Yelp | Personal chef "in name of your city"

COMMUNITY SUPPORTED KITCHEN – ORGANIC TAKE OUT

☐ Three Stone Hearth | www.threestonehearth.com

CREATE AN ONLINE MEAL DELIVERY SCHEDULE FOR FRIENDS AND FAMILY

☐ Lotsa Helping Hands | Care calendar website organizing meals and other help | www.lotsahelpinghands.com

☐ Take Them a Meal | www.takethemameal.com

☐ Meal Train | www.mealtrain.com

DOOR-TO-DOOR FOOD DELIVERY

☐ Caviar | www.trycaviar.com

☐ DoorDash | www.doordash.com

☐ EAT24 | www.eat24.com

☐ GrubHub | www.grubhub.com

☐ MealPal | www.mealpal.com

☐ Uber Eats | www.ubereats.com

☐ Postmates | www.postmates.com

ORGANIC GROCERIES DELIVERED TO YOUR DOORSTEP

☐ Farm Fresh to You | San Francisco | www.farmfreshtoyou.com

☐ Instacart | San Francisco | www.instacart.com

☐ Goodeggs | San Francisco | www.goodeggs.com

☐ bttrventures | Oakland | www.backtotheroots.com

☐ UrbanOrganics | New York | www.urbanorganic.com

☐ Old World Organics | New Jersey | www.greenpeople.org

☐ Door to Door Organics | Colorado www.doortodoororganics.com

☐ Boston Organics | Boston | www.bostonorganics.com

☐ Spud.ca | Vancouver | www.spud.ca

☐ Boxed Greens | Arizona | www.boxedgreens.com

☐ GreenPolkaDotBox | Utah | www.greenpolkadotbox.com

☐ Misfits Market | USA | www.misfitsmarket.com

MEAL BOXED FOOD KIT & DELIVERY TO HOME

☐ Blue Apron | www.blueapron.com

☐ Freshly | www.freshly.com

☐ Green Tiffin | www.greentiffin.com

☐ HelloFresh | www.hellofresh.com

☐ Mealmade | www.mealmade.com

☐ Methodology | www.gomethodology.com

☐ The Purple Carrot | www.purplecarrot.com

☐ Sakara Life | www.sakara.com

☐ Sun Basket | www.sunbasket.com

☐ Thistle | www.thistle.com

☐ Veestro | www.veestro.com

☐ Green Chef | www.greenchef.com

☐ Home Chef | www.homechef.com

JUICE SHOPS WITH FRESH PRESSED JUICE

☐ Joe & The Juice | www.joejuice.com

☐ Juice Shop | www.juiceshop.com

☐ Pressed Juicery | www.pressedjuicery.com

☐ Urban Remedy | www.urbanremedy.com

☐ Google search | Juice shop "near me"

☐ Yelp | Juice shop "in name of your city"

JUICERS FOR IN-HOME DO IT YOURSELF JUICING

☐ Hurom

☐ Breville

☐ Nutri bullet

TEA

☐ LoveJoy's Tea Room | www.lovejoystearoom.com

☐ Samovar Tea Lounge | www.samovartea.com

☐ Stonemill Matcha | www.stonemillmatcha.com

☐ The Scarlet Sage Herb Co. | www.scarletsageherb.com

☐ Google search | Tea "near me"

☐ Yelp | Tea "in name of your city"

WATER

- ☐ Acqua Panna Natural Spring water | www.acquapanna.com
- ☐ Evian | www.evian.com
- ☐ Fiji | www.fijiwater.com
- ☐ Pellegrino | www.sanpellegrino.com
- ☐ Voss | www.voss.com

FASTING

- ☐ The Complete Guide to Fasting by Jason Fung

CBD DRINKS

- ☐ Dram Lemongrass | www.dramapothecary.com
- ☐ GTS Cannabliss Kombucha | www.gtslivingfoods.com
- ☐ Joybird | www.drinkjoybird.com
- ☐ Mary Joe Brand | www.maryjoebrand.com
- ☐ Recess | www.takearecess.com
- ☐ Sprig | www.drinksprig.com
- ☐ Vybes | www.idrinkvybes.com

RESTAURANTS WITH ORGANIC FOCUS

- ☐ Ananda Fuara | www.anandafuara.com
- ☐ Baia | www.matthewkenneycuisine.com
- ☐ Blue Barn | www.bluebarngourmet.com

☐ Bluestone Lane | www.bluestonelane.com

☐ Golden Era Vegan | www.goldeneravegan.com

☐ Gracias Madre | www.gracias-madre.com

☐ Greens Restaurant | www.greensrestaurant.com

☐ Jane | www.itsjane.com

☐ Judahlicious | www.judahlicious.com

☐ Kitava | www.kitava.com

☐ Little Gem restaurant | www.littlegemrestaurant.com

☐ Mixt | www.mixt.com

☐ Native Co | www.nativecosf.com

☐ Next Level Burger San Francisco | www.nextlevelburger.com

☐ Nourish Cafe | www.nourishcafesf.com

☐ Thai Idea Vegetarian Restaurant | thaiideavegetariansf.com

☐ The Plant Cafe Organic | www.theplantcafe.com

☐ Wildseed | www.wildseedsf.com

☐ Google search | Organic restaurant "near me"

☐ Yelp | Organic restaurant "in name of your city"

☐ OpenTable | Make a reservation | www.opentable.com

HEALTHY BAKERY

☐ Arizmendi Bakery | www.arizmendibakery.com

☐ Tartine Bakery | www.tartinebakery.com

☐ The Mill | www.wholesomebakery.com

☐ Wholesome Bakery | www.themillsf.com

☐ Young Kobras | www.youngkobras.com

☐ Google search | Bakery "near me"

☐ Yelp | Bakery "in name of your city"

RETREATS

☐ 1440 Multiversity | Santa Cruz, CA | www.1440.org

☐ Attitudinal Healing International | San Francisco, CA
www.ahinternational.org

☐ Ayurvedic Natural Health Center | Dayton, OH
www.midwestayurveda.com

☐ Commonweal Institute | Bolinas, CA | www.commonweal.org

☐ Dr. McDougall's Health & Medical Center | Santa Rosa, CA
www.drmcdougall.com

☐ Esalen | Big Sur, CA | www.esalen.org

☐ Harmony Hill | Union, WA | www.harmonyhill.org

☐ Hippocrates Health Institute | West Palm Beach, FL
www.hippocratesinstitute.org

☐ Institute for Integrative Nutrition (IIN) | New York, NY
www.bruintegrativenutrition.com

☐ Maharishi Institute of Management | Fairfield, IA
www.mum.edu

☐ Omega Institute for Holistic health | Rhinebeck, NY
www.eomega.org

☐ Shambhala Mountain | Red Feather Lakes, CO
www.shambhalamountain.org

☐ The Raj | Fairfield, IA | www.theraj.com

☐ The UltraWellness Center | Lenox, MA
www.ultrawellnesscenter.com

FINANCIAL SUPPORT

☐ Angels for Shannon | Ease the financial burdens for cancer
patients seeking alternative cancer treatments their insurance will
not cover | www.angelsforshannon.com

☐ GoFundMe | Crowd funding platform | www.gofundme.com

☐ Indiegogo | Crowd funding site | www.indigogo.com

☐ GiveForward | Fundraising tool | www.giveforward.com

☐ Animoto | Video making made easy | www.animoto.com

☐ Wix | Create a website | wix.com

☐ Free will and testiment | www.freewill.com

☐ Legal Zoom | Legal documents | www.legalzoom.com

☐ Aging with Dignity | Improve end-of-life care by making medical
decisions in advance | www.agingwithdignity.org

☐ Five Wishes | Easy-to-use legal advanced directive document that
encompasses medical, personal, emotional and spiritual needs
www.fivewishes.org

SUPPLEMENTS

INDIVIDUAL SUPPLEMENTS:

☐ Adaptocrine

☐ Ashwagandha

☐ Biotin

☐ Calcium D-Glucarate

☐ Calcium Lactate

☐ Cellular Vitality

☐ Chlolenest

☐ Chlorella

☐ Co-Q10 - Ubiquinol

☐ DIM

☐ EPA-DHA 500 Omega 3

☐ Estrium

☐ Folic Acid B12

☐ Glysen

☐ Gotu Kola

☐ HCL Prozyme

☐ HVS Radiation

☐ Inositol Powder

☐ Livton

☐ Lymphonest

☐ MCT oil

- [ ] Methyl SP

- [ ] Micro Minerals

- [ ] Min-Tran

- [ ] Mycosurge

- [ ] Organic coconut oil

- [ ] PhytoMulti

- [ ] PQQ

- [ ] Probilardi

- [ ] Probiotic

- [ ] Repairvite

- [ ] Resveratrol

- [ ] Serenagen

- [ ] Silymarin

- [ ] Tumeric

- [ ] UltraClear Plus

- [ ] Vitamin C

- [ ] Vitamin D3 5000

- [ ] Vitanox

TEETH SUPPORT SUPPLEMENTS

- [ ] BioDent

- [ ] Biost

BRAIN STRENGTH SUPPLEMENTS

☐ Bacopa Brain

☐ Brain Sharpener

SUPPLEMENTS BRANDS

☐ Dr. Frank Lipman | www.bewell.com

☐ Dr. Joseph Mercola | www.mercola.com

☐ Dr. Josh Axe | www.draxe.com

☐ Dr. Mark Hyman | www.drhyman.com

☐ Eco Nugenics | www.econugenics.com

☐ Metagenics | www.metagenics.com

☐ Standard Process | www.standardprocess.com

WEBSITES

BRAIN STRENGTH WEBSITES

☐ Brainhq.com | www.brainhq.com

☐ Luminosity | www.lumosity.com

HEALTH WEBSITES

☐ Blue Zones | Longevity and health | www.bluezones.com

☐ Chris Wark | Natural healing | www.chrisbeatcancer.com

☐ Chris Kresser | Functional medicine | www.chriskresser.com

☐ Cure Joy | Expert advice on healing | www.curejoy.com

- ☐ Dr. Habib Sadeghi | Integrative medicine | behiveofhealing.com

- ☐ Dr. Kelly Turner | Integrative oncology | www.drkellyturner.com

- ☐ Dr. Kevin Conners | Treat the cause | www.connersclinic.com

- ☐ Waylon H. Lewis | Mindful life | www.elephantjournal.com

- ☐ Bani Hari | Food Babe | Food activism | www.foodbabe.com

- ☐ Gabrielle Bernstein | Life coach | www.gabbyb.tv

- ☐ Good Life Project | Build a better life | www.goodlifeproject.com

- ☐ Hay House, Inc. Publishing | Self-help | www.hayhouse.com

- ☐ Hay House Radio | Self-help radio | www.hayhouseradio.com

- ☐ Hay House World Summit | www.youcanhealyourlifesummit.com

- ☐ Erin Elizabeth | Natural health | www.healthnutnews.com

- ☐ Kris Carr | Wellness activist | www.kriscarr.com

- ☐ Martin Seligman | Foundations of positive psychology
  www.authentichappiness.sas.upenn.edu

- ☐ Mary O' Malley | Awakening | www.whatsinthewayistheway.com

- ☐ Michael Roads | Modern mystic | www.michaelroads.com

- ☐ Mike Dooley's | TUT (The Universe Talks) | www.tut.com

- ☐ Mind Body Green | Integrated health | www.mindbodygreen.com

- ☐ Mike Adams | Health Ranger | www.naturalnews.com

- ☐ Brother David Steindl-Rast | Gratitude | www.gratefulness.org

- ☐ Radical remission | Cancer survivors | www.radicalremission.com

- ☐ Sandra Ingerman | Shaman | www.sandraingerman.com

- ☐ Self-development | Inspiration | iheartintelligence.com

☐ Gaia | Consciousness media | www.gaia.com

☐ Tal Ben-Shahar, PhD | Happiness | www.wholebeinginstitute.com

☐ Stephen Dinan | Transformation | www.theshiftnetwork.com

☐ Ty Bolinger | Cancer truths | www.thetruthaboutcancer.com

☐ Well + Good, Llc. | Wellness | www.wellandgood.com

PRODUCTS

☐ Colonic | Enema for detox | www.sawilsons.com

☐ Klean Kanteen | Non-BPA water bottle | www.kleankanteen.com

☐ Meditation | Bracelets | www.meaningtopause.com

☐ Ron Teeguardens | Master herbalist | www.dragonherbs.com

JOURNAL - WRITE THROUGH CANCER

☐ The Five-Minute Journal | www.amazon.com

☐ 5 Minute Daily Gratitude Journal | www.amazon.com

☐ Canvas One Line a Day | www.amazon.com

☐ Journals at Papersource | www.papersource.com

HELP WITH SLEEP

☐ Dr. Michael Breus | Improved sleep | www.thesleepdoctor.com

☐ Tuck | Information on sleep | www.tuck.com

☐ Matthew Walker | Sleep diplomat | www.sleepdiplomat.com

NONPROFITS

☐ Anatara Medicine | Individualized approach to cancer care
www.anataramedicine.com

☐ Breast Cancer Action | Education and activists breast cancer
www.bcaction.org

☐ Breast Cancer Emergency Fund (BCEF) | Financial Assistance
bcef.org

☐ Cancer Finances | How cancer treatment impacts finances
www.cancerfinances.org

☐ Cleaning for a Reason | Free cleaning - cancer treatment
www.cleaningforareason.org

☐ Erik Peper, PhD | BioFeedback and self-regulation
www.biofeedbackhealth.org

☐ Family House | Home for families of children with cancer
familyhouseinc.org

☐ Lolly's Locks | High-quality wigs to cancer patients in need
www.lollyslocks.org

☐ Make-A-Wish Foundation | "Wishes" for children with life-
threatening conditions | www.wish.org

☐ Marion Woodman Foundation | BodySoul work and programs
mwoodmanfoundation.org

☐ Pema Chödrön | Buddhist teacher - mindfulness
www.pemachodronfoundation.org

☐ Project Open Hand | Meals for seniors and adults with disabilities
www.openhand.org

☐ Shanti Project | Support with a life threatening illness
www.shanti.org

☐ The Annie Appleseed Project | Informed treatment choices
www.annieappleseedproject.org

☐ The Cancer Cure Foundation | Research alternative cancer
www.cancure.org

☐ Dr. James Gordon MD | Alternative Medicine | The Center for
Mind Body Medicine | www.cmbm.org

SPIRITUALITY WEBSITES

☐ Anita Moorjani | International speaker NDE cancer survivor
www.anitamoorjani.com

☐ Bernie Siegel, MD | Emotional, physical, spiritual wellness
www.berniesiegelmd.com

☐ Diana Rose | Casa Tour Leaders - John of God
www.celebratinglifeministries.com

☐ Emmanuel Dagher | Spiritual teacher, healer, author
www.emmanueldagher.com

☐ Gregg Braden | www.greggbraden.com

☐ Dr. Kenneth Wapnick | Foundation for a Course in Miracles
Healing power of forgiving love | www.facim.org

☐ Interviews with Ordinary Spiritually Awakening People
www.batgap.com

☐ Anthony Williams | Medical Medium | www.medicalmedium.com

☐ Mooji | Look into who you are | www.mooji.org

☐ Caroline Myss | Workshops | www.myss.com

☐ Near Death Experience Research Foundation | www.nderf.org

☐ Sounds True for wellness | Self-healing | www.soundstrue.com

☐ Oprah Winfrey | Super Soul Sunday | www.oprah.com

☐ Wake Up World | Awakening souls, heart, mind and spirit
www.wakeup-world.com

BOOKS AND MAGAZINES

WELLNESS BOOKS

☐ Authentic Happiness by Martin Seligman

☐ Biology of Belief by Bruce Lipton

☐ Breaking the Habit of Being Yourself by Dr. Joe Dispenza

☐ Chris Beat Cancer by Chris Wark

☐ Deep Medicine by William B. Stewart, MD

☐ Getting Well Again by O. Carl Simonton, MD

☐ Heal Breast Cancer Naturally by Dr. Veronique Desaulniers

☐ Knockout by Suzanne Somers

☐ Medical Medium by Anthony Williams

☐ Radical Remission by Kelly Turner, PhD

☐ Sexy after Cancer by Barbara Musser

☐ Shift Happens by Robert Holden

☐ The Best Friend's Guide to Breast Cancer by Sonja L. Faulkner Ph.D.

☐ The China Study by T. Colin Campbell PhD and Thomas Campbell, MD

☐ Waking the Warrior Goddess by Christine Horner, MD

☐ Women's Bodies, Women's Wisdom by Christiane Northrup, MD

☐ You Can Heal Your Life by Louise Hay

NUTRITION BOOKS

☐ Cancer Free with Food by Liana Werner-Gray

☐ Crazy Sexy Diet by Kris Carr

☐ Grain Brain by Dr. David Perlmutter, MD

☐ Healing with Whole Foods by Paul Pitchford

☐ How Not to Die by Michael Gregor, MD

☐ Stop Fighting Cancer and Start Treating the Cause by Dr. Kevin Conners, MD

☐ The Antianxiety Food Solution by Trudy Scott

☐ The Cancer-Fighting Kitchen: Nourishing, Big Flavor Recipes for Cancer Treatment and Recovery by Mat Edelson and Rebecca Katz

☐ The Detox Prescription by Woodson Merrell

☐ The Great Health Heist by Paul J. Rosen

☐ The Real Truth about Sugar by Dr. Robert Lustig, MD

SPIRITUAL BOOKS

☐ A New Earth Awakening to Your Life's Purpose by Eckhart Tolle

☐ Anatomy of the Spirit by Caroline Myss, PhD

☐ Autobiography of a Yogi by Paramahansa Yogananda

☐ Did You Think to Pray by R.T. Kendall

☐ Dying to be Me by Anita Moorjani

☐ Easy Breezy Prosperity by Emmanuel Dagher

☐ Imagine Heaven by John Burke

☐ Jesus Calling by Sarah Young

- [ ] Journey of Souls by Michael Newton, PhD
- [ ] Living with the Himalayan Masters by Swami Rama
- [ ] Seven Thousand Ways to Listen by Mark Nepo
- [ ] Start Where You Are by Pema Chödrön
- [ ] Talking to Heaven by James Van Praagh
- [ ] The Art of Joyful Living by Swami Rama
- [ ] The Art of Dying by Elizabeth Fenwick and Peter Fenwick
- [ ] The Book of Awakening by Mark Nepo
- [ ] The Essential Wayne Dyer Collection
- [ ] The Gentle Art of Blessing by Pierre Pradervand
- [ ] The Hidden Messages in Water by Dr. Masuro Emoto
- [ ] The Magic Path of Intuition by Florence Scovel Shinn
- [ ] The New Bible Cure for Cancer by Don Colbert, MD
- [ ] The Power of Now by Eckhart Tolle
- [ ] The Tibetan Book of Living and Dying by Sogyal Rinpoche
- [ ] Vaster Than Sky Greater Than Space by Mooji
- [ ] When God & Cancer Meet by Lynn Eib
- [ ] White Fire by Mooji

ENERGY HEALING BOOKS

- [ ] Clear Your Way Home by Marci Baron
- [ ] Wheels of Light Chakras, Auras and the Healing Energy of the Body by Rosalyn Bruyere

CHINESE MEDICINE BOOK

☐ Between Heaven and Earth, A Guide to Chinese Medicine by Harriet Beinfield and Efrem Korngold

CLEAN UP AND DE-CLUTTER BOOK

☐ Life Changing Magic of Tidying Up by Marie Kondo

WRITE THROUGH CANCER BOOK

☐ Writing Your Way Through Cancer by Chia Martin

MAGAZINES

☐ Breast Cancer Wellness | www.breastcancerwellness.org

☐ Common Ground magazine | www.commongroundmag.com

☐ Lion's Roar | www.lionsroar.com

☐ Mindful magazine | www.mindful.org

☐ OM Times | www.omtimes.com

☐ Psychology Today | www.psychologytoday.com

☐ Alternative wellness treatments | www.cancerdefeated.com

☐ Spirituality & Health | www.spiritualityhealth.com

MUSIC FOR HEALING

☐ Binaural beats | Frequencies that promote relaxation, positivity and decrease anxiety | www.binauralbeatsmeditation.com

☐ Health Journeys | Guided imagery and guided meditation www.healthjourneys.com

☐ Kelvin Mockingbird | Native American flute | Album: Wind Child

☐ Michael S. Tyrrell | Vibrational healing | Album: Wholetones

☐ Pandora | Liquid mind, yoga, spa and deuter | www.pandora.com

☐ Solfeggio | Healing frequencies | www.atunedvibrations.com

☐ Tami Briggs | Therapeutic harpist | www.musicalreflections.com

FILMS

☐ Awaken Your Inner Power | www.livelifethemovie.com

☐ The Happy Movie | www.thehappymovie.com

☐ The Sacred Science | www.thesacredscience.com
Nick Polizzi, Three Seed Productions | Eight people with cancer
sent to the Amazon to be healed by Amazonian Shamans.

☐ Food Matters TV | Health & wellness films | www.fmtv.com

☐ Eating Right for Cancer Survival | www.pcrm.org
Neal D. Barnard, MD | Physicians Committee for Responsible
Medicine

☐ Fat Sick and Nearly Dead | www.rebootwithjoe.com | Joe Cross

☐ Food, Inc. | www.foodinc.com

☐ Food Matters | www.fmtv.com

☐ Fork Over Knives | www.forkoverknives.com

☐ Heal | www.healdocumentary.com

☐ Mobilize | www.mobilizemovie.com

☐ Toxic chemicals retardant | www.toxichotseatmovie.com

☐ Explore the U.S. healthcare system | www.escapefiremovie.com

PERSONAL NOTES

☐

☐

☐

☐

☐

☐

☐

☐

☐

☐

☐

PERSONAL NOTES

☐

☐

☐

☐

☐

☐

☐

☐

☐

☐

PERSONAL NOTES

☐

☐

☐

☐

☐

☐

☐

☐

☐

☐

PERSONAL NOTES

- [ ]

- [ ]

- [ ]

- [ ]

- [ ]

- [ ]

- [ ]

- [ ]

- [ ]

- [ ]

- [ ]

Printed in Great Britain
by Amazon

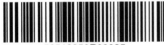